The Merging of the Senses

Cognitive Neuroscience Series
Michael S. Gazzaniga, editor

Cerebral Lateralization: Biological Mechanisms, Associations, and Pathology, Norman Geschwind and Albert M. Galaburda, 1986

Synapses, Circuits, and the Beginning of Memory, Gary Lynch (with commentaries by Gordon M. Shepherd, Ira B. Black, and Herbert P. Killackey), 1986.

The Merging of the Senses, Barry E. Stein and M. Alex Meredith, 1993

The Merging of the Senses

Barry E. Stein and M. Alex Meredith

A Bradford Book
The MIT Press
Cambridge, Massachusetts
London, England

This book was set in Palatino by Achorn Graphic Services Inc.

Library of Congress Cataloging-in-Publication Data

Stein, Barry E.
      The merging of the senses/Barry E. Stein and M. Alex Meredith.
          p.   cm.—(Cognitive neuroscience)
      "A Bradford book."
      Includes bibliographical references and index.
      ISBN 978-0-262--19331-3 (hc : alk. paper), 978-0-262-69301-1 (pb)
      1. Intersensory effects. 2. Perception. 3. Senses and sensation.
I. Meredith, M. Alex. II. Title. III. Series.
      [DNLM: 1. Auditory Perception—physiology. 2. Neurons—
physiology. 3. Superior Colliculus—physiology. 4. Visual
Perception—physiology.   WL 102.5 S819m]
QP441.S73 1993
612.8—dc20
DNLM/DLC
for Library of Congress   92-19598
                                                                                CIP

Contents

Preface

The study of how information from the different senses is integrated in the brain crosses boundaries between a variety of scientific disciplines, such as perceptual psychology, cognitive science, neuroscience, even general biology, and a number of the clinical disciplines such as neurology, neurosurgery, and psychiatry. Thus, we have tried to aim the book at a variety of readers; some may still be students and others will have had very little experience with some of the techniques used in the experiments described here. While some of the information presented has been derived from each of the fields listed above, the primary purpose of this book is to describe the electrophysiological experiments that we have done on single neurons in the central nervous system that code information derived from more than one sensory system. We believe that the manner in which these "multisensory" neurons deal with this information has very direct implications for perception and behavior. These objectives and the general organization of the book are dealt with in more detail in the Introduction.

We would like to extend a special thanks to Nancy London for her willingness to lend her considerable editorial skills to this endeavor. She spent innumerable hours on the many early drafts of each chapter, and served as an excellent consultant with regard to the content and presentation of this material. We are very grateful to her. We would also like to express our gratitude to a number of people who have made helpful comments on various versions of the manuscript. Our thanks to Mark Wallace, Donald Price, Michael Fine, Peter Redgrave, Marc Fariss, Robin Preston, and Werner Graf.

Introduction

Understanding how we perceive the world is of such compelling interest, it is no wonder that so many researchers are involved in studying how the brain codes and analyzes sensory information. To the neuroscientist there is no question that the body and the mind are inextricably bound, and that who we are depends very much on the experiences that are mediated by our sensory systems. But aside from the egocentricity that induces us to engage in the study of the senses, there is also a very real issue of aesthetics involved in this endeavor. For it would be difficult not to be intrigued by the elaborate architecture, remarkable diversity, and exquisite sensitivity of the nervous system's sensory processes and the external organs that serve them.

That evolution should have favored the development of multiple sensory channels by which so many species monitor their external environments hardly seems serendipitous. The coexistence of different sensory modalities significantly enhances an organism's likelihood of survival and the circumstances in which it can flourish. Providing animals with many sources of input that can operate simultaneously or substitute for one another when necessary (e.g., in the dark, auditory and tactile cues must substitute for vision) frees them from many environmental constraints. At the same time, it multiplies their world view, for the different sensory modalities are tuned to different forms of energy, with each giving rise to a qualitatively distinct perceptual experience—a unique "view" of the outside world. There is simply no commonality among the subjective effects or sensory impressions produced, for example, by the sight of a sunset or the sound of a cricket. The perception of hue is unique to the visual system, the perception of pitch is unique to the auditory system, and the perception of tickle is unique to the somatosensory system. The futility of attempting to describe the experience of sight or its specifics, such as color, to a congenitally blind person is sometimes cited as an illustration of the fundamental problem: there is no common ground on which descriptions can be based. Yet, despite the impressive differences in the senses, in certain realms we can relate across them quite readily and are constantly using them in concert without any conscious effort.

Whether this capability is innate or learned is currently a topic of lively debate among developmental psychologists. Some take the position heralded by the Swiss psychologist Jean Piaget that the sensory systems are clearly different and differentiable at birth, and that it is the ability to relate them to one another and to transfer information across them that must be learned through experience. Others suggest that in newborns the sensory modalities are not yet completely differentiated and become so only as a consequence of the individual's experience with the environment. That information can be transferred from modality to modality at very early stages of development is evident from the observation that minutes after birth babies exhibit good visual-tactile intermodal transfer and are capable of imitating certain facial expressions without visual feedback of their own expressions. The inference is that they match what they see to what they "feel." Whether specific experiences during those first few minutes of postnatal life can play any role at all in this cross-modal transfer, whether these infants are matching a visual stimulus to a motor program rather than to how that stimulus looks like it should "feel" tactually, and whether newborns are already capable of apprehending unique qualities in the different senses or actually perceive all senses as the same remain open questions. Not surprisingly, they are also questions that are attracting a good deal of attention among psychologists.

But regardless of whether the newborn brain must learn to distinguish differences between the senses or recognize that there are commonalities among them, it must soon be able to use the *information* it derives from each of them for many of the same purposes (e.g., escaping danger, finding food). In effect, it must be able to evaluate the information processed by the different sensory modalities in ways that are largely independent of the subjective experiences they produce. Therefore, in some ways the sensory information collected by individual modalities is "amodal," or interchangeable among modalities. Such stimulus features as intensity, form, number, and duration are believed to be amodal and are, in fact, transferred readily across modalities. The constancies among amodal stimulus characteristics also provide a basis for perceptual cohesiveness when cues from multiple sensory modalities are present at the same time, thereby facilitating the rapid integration of the information they carry. Such integration is as critical for making sense of the inputs the brain receives from different modalities as it is for interpreting multiple inputs from any single modality. The accuracy and extent of cross-modal matching, cross-modal transfers, and sensory substitutions that depend on these amodal characteristics have been the subjects of fascinating studies in human subjects, and some of these will be discussed here.

Although some modality-specific stimulus characteristics may be largely preserved as the brain sorts out the inputs from many different cues, others are certainly altered. For the world is not perceived as a series of independent sensory experiences in which the integrity of each modality's "snapshot" view is preserved intact in its own location in the brain; rather, there is an interweaving of different sensory impressions through which sensory components are subtly altered by, and integrated with, one another. The product of these integrative processes is perception.

The integration of inputs from different sensory modalities not only transforms some of their individual characteristics, but does so in ways that can enhance the quality of life. Integrated sensory inputs produce far richer experiences than would be predicted from their simple coexistence or the linear sum of their individual products. Aroma and texture are not just independent cues associated with the foods we eat, but, by virtue of their central interaction with inputs from chemical-induced changes on the tongue, are intimately involved in producing the fundamental experience we describe as "taste."

The integration of multiple sensory cues also provides animals with enormous response flexibility, so that the reaction to the presence of one stimulus can be altered by the presence of another. *Context* rather than specific stimulus features now becomes a dominant behavioral determinant, and often even the simplest behaviors require the integration of combinations of environmental stimuli for elicitation. This is particularly well documented in the control of flight in insects, and attentive and orientation behaviors in mammals; some of these examples will be discussed in detail.

Of course, the specific sensory modalities and stimuli that turn out to be "relevant" for producing behavioral responses differ significantly among species, and the degree of dependence on a modality is intimately related to an animal's ecological niche. This makes for fascinating natural diversity: not only do various organisms with the same sensory modalities respond differently to identical stimuli, but different receptors adapt different species to their particular environmental demands. Nevertheless, multisensory integration itself is ubiquitous, and even animals with such seemingly exotic sensory apparatus as an infrared system (pit vipers) or an electroreceptor system (some fish) combine these inputs with those from more commonly represented modalities such as vision to provide an integrated world view.

CONVERGING SENSORY INPUTS

Regardless of the nature of the sensory inputs in any particular species, for the brain to integrate them the different senses must ultimately have access to the same neurons. Indeed, the convergence of different sensory inputs takes place at most levels of the neuraxis. It is especially evident outside the primary projection pathways, but it is by no means unknown within seemingly dedicated unimodal regions.

Both evoked potential and single cell recording techniques have been used to examine the central loci where the convergence of sensory inputs takes place. Such studies have demonstrated its presence in an impressive variety of species. It is evident in unicellular organisms, comparatively simple multicellular organisms such as flatworms, in the higher primates, and at all intervening levels of complexity. In fact, we know of no animal with a nervous system in which the different sensory representations are organized so that they maintain exclusivity from one another. Thus, sensory convergence is unlikely to represent either an epiphenomenon or, in higher animals, a vestige of the plan used in simple organisms, which are forced to make multiple use of a far more limited number of neurons. It seems far more likely that during the evolution of the various sensory systems some mechanisms were preserved and others were introduced so that their combined action could provide information that would be unavailable from their individual operation. Combinations of, for example, visual and auditory cues can enhance one another and can also eliminate any ambiguity that might occur when cues from only one modality are available.

It may seem surprising then, that, in contrast to the extensive efforts being made to understand the methods by which cells in the primary sensory pathways code sensory information and the perceptual consequences of multisensory integration, there has been comparatively little done to understand the neural phenomena that make multisensory integration possible. The paucity of neural data about multisensory integration is due in part to the different strategies researchers have used to explore the functional organization of the nervous system, and also to the inherent difficulties in conducting multisensory studies.

Investigators interested in how neuronal properties subserve a specific sensory modality study neuronal responses to modality-specific stimuli in laboratory conditions that minimize the presence of extraneous stimuli. This is done to limit the possibility that, for example, a nonvisual stimulus might confound the analysis of a neuron's visual responses. The primary objective of these studies is to understand how the functional properties of individual neurons, or groups of neurons, code the parameters of visual stimuli and ultimately give rise to visual sensations, perceptions, and visuomotor responses. Absolute control is exercised over stimulus parameters in a stable environment, so that the only stimulus being varied is the one of interest. In this way, precise quantitative relationships between the properties of a given stimulus and the behavior of a particular neuron are explored. When this sort of analysis is conducted with many hundreds or thousands of neurons, the stimulus features that are coded by neuronal subsets are used to categorize them (e.g., some visually responsive neurons are classified as color-opponent, direction selective, and so on).

This strategy has provided both a wealth of detailed data on how neurons in many structures code sensory stimuli and a good deal of insight into problems of perception and sensorimotor behavior in many sensory modalities. However, nowhere in the objectives of these studies is there included the need to understand how the activity of the neurons classified as, for example, visual, and the sensations and perceptions dependent on their activity are influenced by other sensory modalities. Consequently, it is no surprise that such studies have not contributed much to our understanding of multisensory integration. It was never their purpose. Yet, they have set the high standards necessary for stimulus control in modern sensory neurophysiology. From a practical standpoint, the difficulty of studying how cues are integrated across, rather than within, modalities is some multiple of the number of sensory systems one must examine, a fact that no doubt has daunted many of those who have been interested in the phenomenon of multisensory integration. Yet the same approaches that are used for determining the distribution and response properties of unimodal cells can be used to determine the distribution and characteristics of multisensory cells, and it is with this in mind that we began exploring the sensory convergence patterns and functional consequences of different combinations of sensory stimuli on individual neurons in the mammalian midbrain.

OBJECTIVES AND ORGANIZATION OF THIS BOOK

The primary goal of this book is to examine the neural bases for the brain's ability to integrate the inputs from different sensory systems, and how this integration may be important in producing sensory impressions and behavior—specifically, how these tasks are facilitated by neurons loosely designated as "sensory." Of equal importance, but given far less emphasis here, is the need to give the different sensory modalities ultimate access to the same motoneurons. It is understood that without this kind of convergence on a final common motor output we would never be able to move, for example, a finger in response to a verbal, written, vestibular, or tactile signal. Such concepts are referred to, but are largely beyond the scope of these discussions. Also outside the purview of this book are the interactions that take place outside the central nervous system, in, for example, peripheral skin receptors, such as polymodal nociceptors, which normally respond to a variety of distinctly different physical stimuli (e.g., chemical, mechanical, thermal). Rather, the emphasis here will be on the central integration of cues that are served by receptors such as those in the visual, auditory, and somatosensory systems, whose highly sensitive tuning generally precludes responses to nonadequate stimuli and whose primary projection targets normally function independently of other sensory inputs. Nevertheless, the synthesis of the information contained in these different systems via multisensory integration is often necessary to evoke certain behaviors.

It would simplify matters if we could show that the rules of multisensory integration in the neurons we have been studying pertain directly to sensory systems other than the visual, auditory, and somatosensory systems with which we have dealt in such common laboratory animals as cat and hamster. Unfortunately, we are still ignorant of the nature of the integration across sensory systems in many structures and in most species. Nevertheless, some of the data gathered in several structures and on a wide variety of organisms lead us to believe that the integrative system we have been studying did not arise for the exclusive use of a single population of neurons or one or two laboratory animals, but reflects a general plan that supersedes structure and species.

In large part this book will be a description of the data generated from the select population of neurons that we have studied in the cat superior colliculus and the general "rules" of multisensory integration that have become evident from examining their responses to controlled stimuli. Examining a restricted population of neurons simplifies the task of determining their properties and the likely consequences of the multisensory integration they exhibit. Unfortunately, it also renders somewhat hazardous the task of generalizing from them to neurons in unrelated areas of the brain. However, recent observations in polysensory cortex indicate the generality of the observations in the superior colliculus. These data serve as a preliminary model, or springboard, from which to explore how the brain decides which stimuli from different modalities relate to one another. When used in such fashion, even isolated observations made at the evoked potential or single neuron level in many brain areas of a variety of species can be examined for consistency with data generated in the model neurons. The ultimate objective, of course, is to understand how multisensory integration at the single neuron level, and at the level of groups of neurons, relates to behavior and perception. Although we have already used the data generated from the single neuron to make predictions about attentive and orientation behaviors, thus far our experiments with behavioral techniques have been limited to performance; we have no empirical observations to assess higher cognitive function. It is our hope that the discussions presented here will prompt others to also pursue answers to the extraordinary number of questions that still must be addressed about multisensory integration at neuronal, behavioral, and perceptual levels.

For convenience, the text is divided into four main sections. Part I examines some of the perceptual phenomena in man that illustrate the cooperative (and sometimes conflicting) effects that result when the brain must deal with simultaneous inputs from different sensory modalities. We then begin to explore the neural processes that underlie the integration of multiple sensory inputs by examining what is known about the incidence of sensory convergence at different levels of the nervous system in different species.

Part II is devoted to the organization of the superior colliculus—the model structure that we have been using to understand multisensory integration. This section lays the foundation for the third part by discussing the response properties and organization of the three sensory modalities represented in the superior colliculus: visual, auditory, and somatosensory. It is by examining speculations about the roles played by each sensory respresentation that the organizational parallels and significance of multisensory convergence in this circuit become clear.

Part III deals with the maplike manner in which the different sensory modalities are represented in the superior colliculus and the likely biological significance of their parallel organizations.

Part IV presents what we know about multisensory integration at the level of the single neuron. It begins with an examination of the patterns of sensory convergence, the nature of the interactions among these converging inputs, and the rules of multisensory integration that have been inferred from these observations. The predictive validity of these rules of multisensory integration on attentive and orientation behaviors is then addressed. Included in this section is a discussion of what should (and where possible, what does) happen if some of the normal relationships among the different sensory representations, on which normal multisensory integration is believed to depend, are perturbed. Also included in this section are comparisons among the observations made in the superior colliculus and polysensory cortex, and suggestions for the kinds of data that must be generated in future experiments to more fully appreciate the neural basis of multisensory integration.

I   Intersensory Perceptual Phenomena and Sensory Convergence

The literature dealing with multisensory integration in human perception (generally referred to as "intersensory" or "intermodal" rather than "multisensory") has a history that antedates the formal establishment of its mother discipline, psychology. Similarities and differences in the subjective experiences produced by each of the senses, their ability to influence one another, and their accuracy in reflecting events in the external world have been subjects of more than passing interest to philosophers since at least the time of Aristotle (it seems quite unlikely that pre-Aristotelian man had no thoughts on this matter, but dating things to Aristotle gives them the provenance sufficient for most purposes).

Although psychology now has the firmest claim on the study of perception, contributions to the understanding of intersensory influences on perception have come from a variety of other disciplines, most notably philosophy and neurology, and now neuroscience. The field has, in fact, become so large that subfields have subfields; for example, the literature dealing with the development of intersensory influences is often divided into studies of older or younger infants. Consequently, no attempt is made here to present a comprehensive review of this body of knowledge.

The purpose of chapter 1 is to provide a selective discussion of examples of human perceptual phenomena that are currently being investigated and that may relate to the physiological studies to be discussed in later sections. Of primary concern are observations that the use of one sensory system can influence (e.g., enhance, degrade, change) perception via another sensory system, and that information can be transferred readily across modalities so that they may substitute for one another. Hence, the section will deal with the intersensory consequences of modality-specific stimuli. The measure of these effects is generally behavioral when dealing with human subjects, although evoked potentials do give us some insight into what is happening in the central nervous system during such tests. Evoked potentials in human subjects also form a bridge to what has been done at the physiological level in animals. Although the primary subject matter of the remainder of this volume is derived from studies of multisensory interactions at the single neuron level in animals, the ultimate objective of these studies is to help understand the neural basis of intersensory perceptual phenomena in man. The reader may rest assured that this objective will not be fully realized here, but juxtaposing the results from perceptual and physiological investigations emphasizes the long-term goal. This juxtaposition may also provide some interesting parallels among disciplines and insights into the design of future experiments in both animals and humans to begin bridging the very real gap that presently exists between perceptual and physiological studies. These last statements reflect a perspective that should be made explicit: the principles of multisensory convergence and interaction based on single neuron and evoked potential studies in animals are applicable to the understanding of human perception.

Because the integration of multiple sensory inputs takes place in virtually all organisms and requires that these inputs converge somewhere in the central nervous system, chapter 2 is devoted to examining the widespread nature of multisensory convergence at different levels of the nervous system in various species. Speculations about possible evolutionary changes that took place in multisensory representations during the evolution of multicellular organisms are presented, as are some regarding possible changes in the thalamus and cortex during mammalian evolution.

1   Intersensory Perceptual Phenomena in Humans

THE VENTRILOQUISM EFFECT

At one time or another almost all of us have been charmed by the skill of an effective ventriloquist. You don't quite suspend your belief that wooden heads can't talk, and you always know which one is the dummy and which one is not, but because the dummy's lips, eyes, and head are moving and the ventriloquist's aren't, you experience the voice as coming from the dummy (figure 1.1). This entertainer's trick actually says more about the audience than the performer, because the experience is due less to his capability to throw his voice than to the dominance of some sensory cues over the perception of others. The ventriloquist's task is to make the experience as compelling as possible by eliminating extraneous stimuli, directing your attention to the dummy, ensuring that the dummy's lips move in approximate synchrony with his speech, and keeping a minimal distance between his mouth and the dummy's. Ultimately, however, the illusion that the dummy is speaking depends on the interaction among the different sensory inputs in the perceiver.

In psychology, the term "ventriloquism effect" (Howard and Templeton 1966) refers to the broader phenomenon of intersensory bias, where, for example, vision can influence judgments about proprioception and audition, proprioception can bias auditory judgments, and so on (e.g., Held 1955; Pick et al. 1969; Thurlow and Rosenthal 1976; Shelton and Searle 1980; Welch and Warren 1980; Warren et al. 1981). The magnitude of intersensory bias and the dominant modality depend on how compelling or real each individual cue is (Welch and Warren 1986). The cues can be weighted very differently when combined with one another, and it is their final integrated product that determines the perception of, and the reaction to, an event.

Generally, in intersensory influences, the visual modality predominates. That is, unless there are dramatic differences in the intensities of different stimuli, the visual effect on the information generated in most other sensory systems is greater than their effect on visual perception. The ventriloquism effect is but one example.

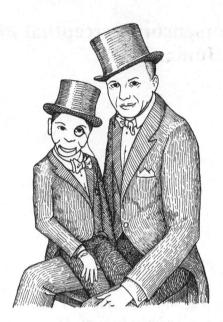

Figure 1.1 The ventriloquism effect. The ventriloquist "throws his voice" by minimizing his own movements so that the only visual cues the audience can associate with speech come from the dummy. This says less about the ventriloquist's skill than about how strong visual-auditory intersensory biases are in the audience.

The power of visual stimuli on other sensory experiences is perhaps best illustrated by the effects achieved in some films shown in specialized theaters and planetariums. By mimicking the visual cues associated with a bush plane navigating through a rugged mountain range or one of the roller coaster rides so attractive to terror-seeking children, they initiate not only very real vestibular sensations, but a wide range of interesting visceral sensations as well. One experience with these visually evoked vestibular (and accompanying gastrointestinal) changes is quite sufficient to dramatize the power of intersensory biases. Although it will not be immediately apparent from such an experience in the theater, visual-vestibular intersensory effects can be bidirectional if one has control over the salience of the various cues. For example, if visual cues are minimal in situations in which vestibular and visual cues are discordant, the vestibular influences will now dominate. In a dark room one can judge the orientation of an illuminated line quite accurately even though there is no visible background. But if the same judgments are made during or immediately after centrifugal rotation, the line appears to be tilted (figure 1.2). These judgments, then, are based at least in part on the perceived orientation of the body in relation to the rest of the world (e.g., gravity) via signals from the vestibular system. Illusory changes in the judgment of line orientation seem to be achieved by a variety of different actions as long as they somehow alter vestibular system function. Even allowing the vestibular system to adapt to a maintained tilt of the head and/or body will interfere with accurate

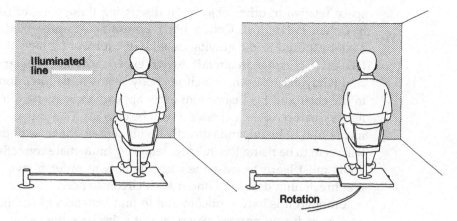

Figure 1.2 Visual-vestibular interaction. When visual cues are minimal (darkened room), the orientation of an illuminated line appears to change to match the effects of rotation on the perception of the body's vertical axis.

visual judgments of line orientation (Clark and Graybiel 1966; Wade and Day 1968).

These same mechanisms of vestibular activation also change auditory perceptions, altering the apparent location of a sound (Graybiel and Niven 1951; Lackner 1974a,b). However, as soon as there is enough visual information available to accurately judge one's body position, the visual cues become dominant; now dependence on vestibular inputs or judgments based on gravity are lowered, and the visual tilt illusion and mislocation of auditory cues are ameliorated significantly, and may even disappear.

The effect of gravity on visual perception is of more than theoretical interest to pilots and astronauts, who regularly experience major shifts in the gravitational-inertial field during take-offs, landings, changes in acceleration, and space flight. For them an appreciation of the effect of conflicting information from internal receptors (i.e., proprioceptive cues) and visual cues is critical for survival. For example, in a zero-gravity environment the eyes shift upward and objects appear to be lower than they actually are. In a hypergravity environment the exact opposite occurs. In both cases the individual is unaware of the shift in the resting position of the eyes, and could make disastrous choices if he makes judgments based on his perceived location in space or his location relative to other objects. Similar perceptual changes can be induced without actual eye movements, by simply changing the proprioceptive cues initiated in the extraocular or neck muscles by gently vibrating them (Roll et al. 1991). Even vibrating the muscles on only one side of the neck makes it appear as if a target in a darkened room is displaced contralaterally or is moving in that direction (Biguer et al. 1988). All of these data remind us that multiple cues are normally synthesized when making judgments of one's position and perspective in space relative to other objects. In discussing these sorts of issues (see B. Cohen 1981; M.M. Cohen 1981), an example is presented in which a pilot exposed to the gravitational-inertial forces of a high acceleration take-off (e.g., from an aircraft carrier) experiences an "oculogravic" illusion (Graybiel 1952), in which his body seems to be tilted too far back in the chair and his instrument array appears to be rising too fast. The illusory nature of the experience will be obvious if he checks his instruments. But, if he depends directly on his senses, the nose of the aircraft will seem to be rising too quickly, requiring immediate corrective action. Pilots must learn to trust their instruments in order to avoid making life-threatening decisions under such circumstances.

Although it is hardly uncommon to find instances of conflicting sensory cues during normal experience, it is because the sensory systems have evolved to work in concert that misperceptions occur when multisensory cues conflict. The general synergy between the visual and auditory systems is particularly evident in the perception of speech. Being in a room with significant background noise will make it difficult to understand someone speaking in normal tones, but seeing the speaker's face will make it far easier to understand what is being said. A recent neuromagnetic study by Sams and colleagues (1991) indicates that the sight of lip movement actually modifies activity in the auditory cortex. By whatever mechanism the visual cue actually enhances the processing of auditory inputs, it is the functional equivalent of altering the signal-to-noise ratio of the auditory stimulus by 15–20 decibels (Sumby and Pollack 1954). *Correctly* perceiving what is said depends on being able to properly visualize the movements that give rise to speech. Experimental support for this idea comes from studies in which nonmatching visual and auditory cues in speech are combined. The results are interesting products known as auditory-visual illusions, and are discussed in an article entitled "Hearing lips and seeing voices" (McGurk and MacDonald 1976). An example of such an illusion occurs when one hears "ba-ba" but sees the mouth form "ga-ga" and perceives the sound "da-da." Perhaps it is not so strange, then, when someone says: "I can't hear you, I don't have my glasses on."

The synergy of visual and proprioceptive systems is evident in the impairment of spatial judgments by the visual system after destruction of the vestibular apparatus or owing to lesions or inflammation of neck muscles (see B. Cohen 1981). Perhaps this is a result of disrupting the gaze system, the system in which the integration of visual and proprioceptive cues is most heavily used to coordinate eye and head movements. To maintain fixation on a moving visual target or on a stationary target when the head moves, inputs from movement sensors (e.g., the vestibular system), vision, and somatosensory receptors (e.g., neck and extraocular proprioceptors) are combined to determine the proper compensatory responses to send back to the muscles controlling these peripheral systems. Consequently, while compensatory eye movements could be induced with either visual or vestibular cues alone, the information from both is used in an interdependent fashion.

Intersensory calculations are made possible, in large part, by the great numbers of common neural targets throughout relevant parts of the vestibular system, where different inputs interact directly. One such target is the mossy fiber input system to the cerebellum and another involves cerebellar neurons (e.g., Purkinje cells) themselves. Some mossy fibers already carry multisensory (e.g., visual and vestibular) as well as oculomotor information, while others carry only unisensory information about visual image slip (the difference between visual fixation and the actual location of the image on the retina). The convergence and interaction of inputs onto flocculus neurons of the cerebellum allows for the initiation of corrective signals, which are sent to the muscles to produce movements that keep the image stabilized on the retina for proper tracking (e.g., Noda 1981; Waespe et al. 1981). Interactions among visual and vestibular inputs in the control of gaze have received a great deal of attention, and a series of excellent discussions is available elsewhere (see Henn et al. 1980; B. Cohen 1981; Berthoz and Jones 1985; Cohen and Henn 1988).

REACTION TIME AND EVOKED POTENTIALS

Cooperative interactions among sensory modalities are also apparent during generalized reactions to an event. Here the functional synergy among sensory systems carrying concordant information is evident as an increase in overall reaction speed, as well as in the physiological processes that signal the presence of the stimulus complex. It is well known that our reactions to an auditory stimulus are faster than to a visual stimulus. Generally this difference is on the order of 40–60 msec and is largely due to the longer stimulus processing time in the retina as compared to the inner ear. However, when a visual stimulus precedes an auditory stimulus by the difference in visual-auditory processing time so that the two inputs converge simultaneously, the reaction time to the stimulus becomes significantly shorter than it was to either stimulus alone. Most investigators seem to agree that such bisensory stimuli speed up reactions (e.g., Hershenson 1962; Morrell 1968a,b, 1972; Bernstein et al. 1969; Andreassi and Greco 1975; Posner et al. 1976; Gielen et al. 1983; but see Colavita 1974; Colavita and Weisberg 1979), but there is some disagreement on the mechanisms by which this is effected. Since higher intensity stimuli generally produce faster reactions than do lower intensity stimuli regardless of modality, some believe that the explanation lies in a central summing of the energies of the two stimuli (presumably analagous to a multisensory interaction). While not denying this possiblity, Nickerson (1973) suggests that the same observations might be explained by invoking a "preparation enhancement," or alerting effect of one stimulus on another, while still others believe that both mechanisms are necessary to explain the reported observations (Bernstein 1970; also see Welch and Warren 1986). The presence of an enhanced physiological response to combinations of different sensory stimuli at the single neuron level, which will be discussed in subsequent chapters, lends greatest support to the presence of a central interaction of sensory inputs, and this is further supported by evoked potential data.

In experiments that combined reaction time measures with evoked potential recordings, Andreassi and Greco (1975) showed that presenting a visual stimulus before an auditory stimulus speeds up a subject's reactions to the auditory cue but is, of course, incapable of increasing the speed of processing in the peripheral sensory organs, the speed with which axons conduct the input from the ear to the brain, or the *initial* processing of the input within the central nervous system. Thus, the evoked potential latencies for visual plus auditory stimuli were not shorter than those for the auditory stimulus alone, but the amplitude of the evoked potential to the combined stimulus was significantly greater than to either stimulus alone. Similar findings with simultaneous visual and auditory stimuli have been provided by Costin and coworkers (1991). These experimenters note that while the combination of stimuli enhances the early evoked responses to these sensory inputs and shortens reaction time, the appearance of a late potential depends on their combination and is thus multisensory.

While it may not seem surprising that two stimuli can produce a larger evoked potential than one, often two stimuli of the same modality inhibit one another or fail to summate as expected (e.g., see Walter 1964; Davis 1968; Shipley 1980). These data are consistent with a central interaction of stimuli from different sensory modalities, and with the idea that increasing the magnitude of the evoked potential increases the salience of a stimulus. Presumably the increased salience of the stimulus quickly renders it far less ambiguous to the subject, so that he now responds more quickly. The covariance of increased stimulus salience and magnitude of the evoked potential with multisensory stimuli is supported by the observation that unlike normal children, mentally retarded and dyslexic children have greater difficulty dealing with multisensory stimuli than with unimodal stimuli, and their evoked potentials show a proportionately lower summation of multisensory stimuli than do normals (Shipley 1980).

Additional data supporting the idea that multisensory evoked potentials reflect the interaction of sensory cues come from a variety of studies in animals which will be discussed in the next chapter. Although it will not be an exhaustive survey of the number of places in the brains of every species examined where inputs from different sensory modalities converge and their functional inputs intermingle, even this truncated list is impressively long. Given the number of such multisensory areas in the brain, it might seem surprising that we are not far more aware of intersensory influences than we are. Normally, however, we pay little attention to the interactions that take place in the confluence of sensory cues we encounter, and we tend to act as if the senses are quite independent of each other. But for some, the daily experience with sensory stimuli is quite different.

SYNESTHESIA

A particularly provocative but poorly understood syndrome, in which the sensory systems appear to be far less distinguished from one another than is generally assumed, is the synesthetic experience. Synesthesia literally means "joining the senses," and it is believed by some to reflect ". . . an involuntary joining in which the real information of one sense is accompanied by a perception in another sense" (Cytowic 1989). The example of sonogenic synesthesia, in which music provokes intense visual experiences or cutaneous paraesthesias, has been known for well over 100 years (Critchley 1977; Henson 1977), and isolated cases of visually evoked auditory sensations were reported in the 1700s. During the nineteenth century it was fashionable among those in polite society to have had synesthetic experiences. As a result, there were many clinical and scientific reports of synesthetic experiences, but because there was no way to evaluate their physical bases, it was almost impossible to differentiate among those who simply wanted to be fashionable, those whose symptoms reflected psychiatric disorders, and those properly classified as synesthetic. As a consequence, serious inquiry into synesthesia was abandoned during the first half of this century. It is currently enjoying a resurgence of interest among neurologists and developmental psychologists, and it is now impossible to avoid this topic in any discussion of multisensory integration.

Recently, Cytowic (1989) presented a fascinating, extensive list of detailed case reports of synesthesia in a volume dedicated to the topic; one example consistent with his description is presented in figure 1.3 (also see Marks 1978). Synesthetes appear to cut across a variety of social milieus and personalities, and some of their perceptual descriptions are remarkably rich in detail. Unfortunately, it is difficult to interrelate the variety of subjective experiences that the patients described to the author as being characteristic of their synesthetic episodes, and there are still no reliable data to help determine whether they share similar neurological etiologies. Furthermore, statements like "synesthesia may be a remnant of how early mammals perceived their world" and may occur when "the cortex briefly ceases to function in the modern manner" (p. 176) strain the reader's credulity. Still, there is little doubt that the patients have compelling sensory experiences in one modality that are triggered by stimuli in another (an amusing example included in a book aimed at the general reader is that of a woman who tasted baked beans

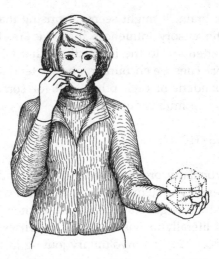

Figure 1.3 Synesthesia. For this synesthete, a particular taste always induces the sensation of a particular geometric form in her left hand.

every time she heard the word "Francis"; see Ackerman 1990). More-over, subjects have had these experiences for as long as they can re-member, the episodes are never volitional and are stable over a lifetime. The more unreliable reports have been culled by the author, and it may be a bit hasty to dismiss the remainder out of hand as due to the overac-tive imaginations of those in the patient population.

Accepting synesthetic experiences as real is not the same as accepting the premise that they represent a "confusion" of the senses as is so often claimed. At this point one should not be too quick to eliminate a more conservative explanation, that the synesthesias reflect a fusion of sensory experiences via association phenomena, in which independent groups of neurons are activated in close temporal proximity to one an-other via long chains of synaptic connections. Their concurrent activity can produce a perceptual synthesis after repeated pairings much like any other conditioned experience (one example of which is cross-modality associations based on shared meaning; see Marks 1975, 1978).

A number of compelling examples of the power and long-lasting na-ture of intersensory association is provided by Kohler (1964) from his experiments in which vision was distorted in various ways by wearing different kinds of spectacles. In one case a subject wore spectacles in which the left halves were blue and the right halves were yellow. When he looked left everything appeared to be blue, when he looked right everything was yellow. After a while the subject reported a subjective fading of both colors, but removal of the spectacles produced aftereffects which, as is usual with such illusions, were complementary to the initial sensations. Now a gaze shift to the left produced a heightened sensitiv-ity to yellow, while gaze shifts to the right heightened sensitivity to blue. Somehow the kinesthetic cues associated with one set of neck and eye muscle inputs became associated with one color, and another set of neck and eye signals with the other color. Despite the fact that the colored spectacles produced nonsensical color experiences and were worn for only 20 days, the associations formed during that time produced aftereffects that were evoked immediately with the appropriate movement and were still evident 11 days after removing the spectacles.

On the other hand, the synesthetic experiences are also consistent with the sort of sensory mixing (confusion?) that would be predicted from a simple survey of the number of brain areas in which different modalities converge on the same neurons. It might not be surprising to find that one dominant input directly evokes secondary sensations in other modalities via such multisensory neurons. While some lean heavily toward the former explanation, Cytowic would likely favor a more extreme version of the latter. But, since few of us would be classified as synesthetes despite the fact that we are all prone to associations among modalities and presumably all of us have multisensory neurons, neither alternative provides a wholly satisfying explanation of these reports.

While the absence of an acceptable neural explanation of these experiences is unfortunate, it should have little impact on an appreciation of the phenomenon itself. Whether due to association or the activation of multisensory neurons, synesthesia reflects the rich multisensory perceptual experiences that appear to be quite common in select individuals. To some, the rarity of the synesthete represents less of an oddity per se than an individual who retains a normal neonatal state for an abnormally long period. In other words, the synesthete is believed to be someone experiencing the effects of arrested sensory development.

DEVELOPMENT AND DIFFERENTIATION OF THE SENSES

Although the primary sensory pathways are quite advanced at birth, some investigators believe that their influences in the central nervous system are poorly differentiated from one another—more specifically, that the different senses form a primitive unity (e.g., von Hornbostel 1938; Ryan 1940; Gibson 1966; Bower 1977; Marks 1978; Turkewitz and Mellon 1989) and one must learn to differentiate among them. This view is quite different from that of Piaget (1952) and Helmholtz (1884/1968), who believed that the senses are separate from one another at birth and that postnatal experience in their use is required before they can be interrelated. There is the appearance of a logical inconsistency in the primitive unity hypothesis. The capability to learn to differentiate among the senses assumes that there already exists some distinguishable characteristics in the sensations they produce. Proponents would point to the possibility that to the infant these differences may already exist, but are evoked collectively so that their separate identities are not immediately apparent without experience. Thus, an initiating stimulus produces "sensations (that) spill from one sensory system into another" (Maurer and Maurer 1988, p. 164). The unity is then due to evoking a complex of different sensations at nearly the same time. In addition, the postulate does not preclude a gradual development of the physical system coincident with the experience of using it.

In this view every infant is synesthetic, although most gradually grow out of it. The evidence for infant synesthesia seems to be based on inference, on the equivalence judgments made by them when different sensory stimuli are presented, and on the comparatively broad territories invaded by unimodal evoked potentials in infants—a shaky base for such a far-reaching postulate. Nevertheless, some of the recent observations made in neonates do question long-held assumptions about the gradual development of certain intersensory capabilities, and make one wonder whether explanations based on traditional association phenomena are adequate to explain them.

Perhaps the most dramatic example that gives rise to such questions is that of Meltzoff and colleagues (Meltzoff and Moore 1977, 1983a,b), who showed that within minutes of birth babies could imitate the investigator's facial expression, as shown in figure 1.4.

In these studies the sight of the investigator sticking his tongue out led the babies to stick out their own tongues. Yet the babies had never had the opportunity to see their own faces or tongues, and therefore could not have formed concrete visual-visual associations. Similarly, babies imitated the investigator's lip-protrusion and mouth opening movements. These findings have been interpreted by some as consistent with infant synesthesia, and it has been suggested that infants match what they see to tactile sensations that are evoked *directly* by the visual stimulus (Maurer and Maurer 1988). Meltzoff himself is somewhat more conservative, never suggesting that the two experiences are undifferentiated, but that infants have an innate ability to make judgments based on some equivalent, presumably amodal, features among modalities (see Gibson 1966; Jones 1981; Gibson 1983; Spelke 1987; Rose 1990; see the section on Cross-Modal Matching presented below for a discussion of amodal stimuli).

Facial imitation is thought to represent the infant's matching of what it sees to some equivalent features of the proprioceptive signals that it feels while trying to mimic, a process referred to by Meltzoff as "active intermodal mapping" (why an infant has the slightest inclination to imitate the investigator at all is a puzzling question itself). The observation that infants will visually explore the same pacifier they have just sucked on (different shapes were used) rather than a pacifier of a different shape, even though they were not allowed to see either of them until the visual test was performed, was taken as consistent with this postulate (Meltzoff 1990).

These kinds of observations put a crimp in the idea that facial imitation does not take place until 1 year of age or more (Piaget 1962), and

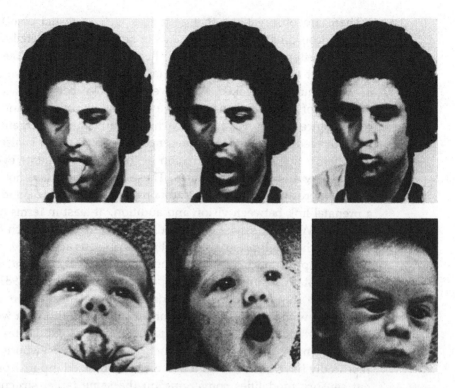

Figure 1.4 Infant imitation. These photographs from videotaped recordings of 2- to 3-week-old infants show that very young children are capable of matching visual cues with their own tactile/proprioceptive sensations to imitate tongue protrusion (*left*), mouth opening (*center*), and lip protrusion (*right*). (From Meltzoff, A.N. and Moore, M.K. 1977. Imitation of facial and manual gestures by human neonates. Science 198: 75–78. Copyright AAAS)

challenged those who describe imitative behavior as based on instrumental learning theories. It is, perhaps, no surprise that the initial report of these findings (Meltzoff and Moore 1977) met with some aggressive criticisms (e.g., Anisfeld et al. 1979; Abravanel 1981), but not because the authors claimed that infants exhibit intersensory integration: this same claim was made previously (Bower et al. 1970; Aronson and Rosenbloom 1971) and even shown for the imitation of facial gestures (Gardner and Gardner 1970). The criticisms were made because these capabilities were claimed to appear very early in life. The follow-up studies done by these investigators moved the appearance date from weeks after birth to minutes after birth and pointed to an innate capability for detecting at least some forms of cross-modal equivalence. Although some feel that these data and interpretations are still somewhat controversial (Turkewitz and Mellon 1989) and some investigators have had difficulty in demonstrating some of these effects in young infants (Spelke 1987; Meltzoff and Kuhl 1989; Rose 1990), a number of the observations have now been replicated elsewhere (see Meltzoff 1990 for a complete list of replications).

There are observations that sound as well as visual objects evoke spatially coordinated eye movements in neonates (for a detailed discussion see Butterworth 1981). This has been known for some time in older infants, but now is being examined far earlier. There is at least one case in which auditory-evoked eye movements have been claimed within moments of birth, and in another a congenitally blind infant showed convergence of the eyes to approaching sounds and divergence of the eyes to receding sounds. The presence of a visual target is also known to enhance the spatial coordination of the eye movements evoked by an auditory stimulus in neonates. These observations are not explainable by mere arousal effects or traditional learning theories, and suggest a prenatal link between vision and audition, at least in terms of spatial relations. Whether innate or immediately acquired, any such link that enhances the localization of a stimulus has obvious advantages and may be "an adaptive mechanism that lends coherence to, but is independent of, the content of any particular experience" (Butterworth 1981, p. 49).

The idea that links between modalities are established prenatally is consistent with modern neuroanatomical findings, although we do not yet understand much about the synaptic or physiological consequences of multisensory convergence at such early stages. Newborn animals repeatedly have been shown to have well-organized inputs from different sensory modalities converging on the same target structure. Presumably these inputs are also synapsing onto some of the same neurons. Indeed, at an anatomical level, the fetal and newborn brains of some animals may be thought of as more multisensory than those of the same animals when they are adults, because they exhibit multisensory convergence in structures known to be unimodal at maturity. The "nonappropriate" inputs to these structures normally are lost during early stages of maturation unless extraordinary surgical means are taken to preserve them (Frost 1984; Innocenti and Clarke 1984; Asanuma et al. 1988; Roe et al. 1990). Furthermore, in some species, providing patterned visual input earlier in development than normal—for example, by separating the eyelids in mammals (Kenney and Turkewitz 1986; Turkewitz and Mellon 1989) or extending the heads of bird embryos from their shells (Gottlieb et al. 1989; Lickliter 1990)—affects their use of other sensory systems. Thus, the idea that there are intersensory links established prenatally is a more conservative view than supposing that all such connections are established after parturition. Experience seems to play its primary roles in determining which convergence patterns will survive and how the different inputs will be weighted functionally (see chapter 12).

The superior colliculus is one of the sites in the central nervous system in which a convergence of visual, auditory, and somatosensory inputs occurs (Stein 1984b). This has been demonstrated repeatedly in many species. The anatomical projections from multiple sensory systems already are evident at parturition, and physiological studies have shown that multisensory neurons become functional quite early in postnatal life and are retained throughout adulthood. Because many of these neurons also project to areas of the brain stem controlling eye movements, the finding that auditory stimuli will evoke coordinated eye movements in newborn children and in congenitally blind children is not terribly surprising. It had been postulated earlier that eye movements might be evoked soon after birth in altricial animals, who are virtually blind at this time, by somatosensory and auditory stimuli that are able to drive the multisensory output neurons of the superior colliculus (Stein et al. 1980; also see Stein et al. 1973). Because the visual, somatosensory, and auditory representations in the superior colliculus share the same maplike representations (see chapter 6), nonvisually evoked eye movements would be directed toward the source of the stimulus, just as they would if evoked visually. However, since auditory receptive fields are generally larger than visual receptive fields here, one would expect the eye movements to auditory stimuli to be less accurate than those to visual targets, an effect that has been noted when the accuracy of eye movements to auditory and visual stimuli has been compared in human infants (Spelke 1987) and in cats (Hartline and Northmore 1986).

CROSS-MODAL MATCHING

Once one begins dealing with older infants and especially adults, the disputes about whether equivalence judgments among modalities can be made and whether information can be transferred across modalities are no longer prevalent. This does not mean that controversy in these areas disappears (it doesn't), only that the nature-nurture questions become less pressing and there is little disagreement that intersensory integration is a fundamental characteristic of normal perception. The mechanisms on which intersensory judgments are based remain an area of fertile speculation.

The best known and most frequently studied intersensory phenomenon is that of cross-modal matching. Cross-modal matching is using information obtained through one sensory modality to make a judgment about an equivalent stimulus from another modality. A typical cross-modal task is shown in figure 1.5 and involves seeing an object (such as a ball) and then using somatosensory (i.e., haptic) cues to judge which of a variety of objects is most similar to the one seen. Unless the judgments required are particularly subtle, there is no difficulty in this sort of task for most normal adults and older children. Even very young children exhibit the ability to match haptically and visually explored objects (Abravanel 1981) and can detect incongruities in matches of visual and auditory stimuli (Lyons-Ruth 1977).

While cross-modal matching is clearly an intersensory phenomenon, and may involve multisensory neurons, one could make a case that it has little to do with the integration of inputs from different modalities

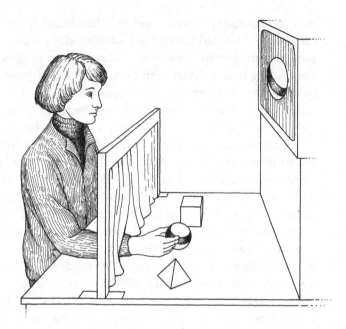

Figure 1.5 Cross-modal matching. The visual features of an object can be readily matched with those evoked by tactile (haptic) cues.

per se, and that multisensory areas of the brain need not play any special role in this process. The judgments of equivalence across modalities could depend on the individual inputs being held in the central nervous system in modality-specific form, so that they are independent of one another but still may be accessed by another neural pool (Wallach and Averback 1955; Ettlinger and Wilson 1990).

It is also possible that the various modality-specific inputs are converted into the reference scheme of a single modality (one could engage in a semantic argument about whether the involvement of such a conversion means that all later processes should be referred to as multisensory, but this becomes too tortured an argument to be productive). Generally, those in favor of the single reference scheme believe that spatial information is encoded in visual coordinates. This belief is based, in part, on demonstrations that congenitally blind people and those who are sighted (or blind but were previously sighted) perceive tactile information in very different ways (Pick 1974). In some cases observations with normally sighted subjects also lead to this conclusion. In an experiment conducted by Natsoulas and Dubanoski (1964), the subject reported that a *b* traced on his forehead was a *d*. The same letter *b* traced on the back of the subject's head was correctly identified. Apparently the subject evaluated the letter on the basis of what it would look like if seen, and this was confirmed by the subject verbally.

Alternatively, sensory information may be held in some amodal form, where interactions among inputs would still play little or no role. From an experiential perspective there appears to be a simple way of constructing well-defined amodal scales through which intersensory comparisons can be made (although primitive scales are likely to be present at birth). All stimuli, regardless of modality, can be ranked according to a continuous scale in terms of such physical characteristics as their intensity, size, number, spatial location, and duration. One can then scale the softest to the loudest sound along the same ten-point analogue scale as the dimmest to the brightest light, or the softest to the most forceful pressure on the fingertips. The scale then becomes a common metric and can be used to make equivalence judgments among modalities. This common metric can even be used to make equivalence judgments about things like desire, or expectation, or pain (Stevens 1975; Price 1988). A typical visual analogue scale, in which the scale is organized to look like a ruler, and in this case is used to rate the intensity of a noxious stimulus, is shown in figure 1.6.

The fact that amodal coding of information can actually take place in the brain has already been demonstrated at the level of the single neu-

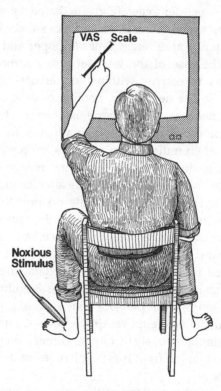

Figure 1.6 The visual analogue scale (VAS). In this case a noxious stimulus to the foot is being scaled. The subject indicates a point along the scale (left is lowest) that corresponds to his judgment of the relative intensity of the stimulus. All sensory stimuli can be ranked from minimum to maximum along this common metric. The scale can then be used to make judgments of equivalence among the different senses. (Modified from Stein et al. 1989)

ron. Some neurons in higher level visual cortex (i.e., V4) are tuned to specific line orientations, and will respond selectively to this orientation whether it is presented as a visible line or as a bar that is felt with the hand but not seen (Maunsell et al. 1989). Consequently, the information coded in these neurons is not specific for a given sensory modality, and is amodal. However, even if such scales were used, the actual mechanism that one would use to relate one modality to another remains obscure.

It is not yet possible to choose among these possible alternatives in seeking the neural library used as *the* basis for cross-modal matching, or even to decide if only one scheme is relevant. Indeed, all the schemes outlined above (and others, such as coding sensory inputs in motor coordinates) might coexist in different areas of the brain or even in different dimensional capabilities of the same neurons, and all may be used in concert.

This last possibility may seem particularly odd. But the same neuron can be involved in multiple circuits and have multiple roles, depending on the particular complex of stimuli and the organism's current state. State-dependent cues (e.g., mediated by neuromodulators) can alter a neuron's membrane characteristics so that it can be recruited into different circuits at different times (Hooper and Moulins 1989).

In the case of the multisensory neuron it is possible for the same neuron to convey within- and across-modality information simultaneously. For despite the pooling of different sensory inputs onto common neurons, the unique character of these inputs need not be obliterated. Each modality maintains its own spatial representation, even when multiple sensory cues are present simultaneously. An auditory cue does not alter the visual receptive field of an auditory-visual neuron, nor does the visual cue alter its auditory receptive field. In other words, their combined inputs do not disrupt their individual spatial representations. Nevertheless, in the presence of multiple sensory stimuli striking interactions take place, and these interactions produce a dramatic enhancement or depression of the overall level of activity evoked from the neuron. These data, therefore, are consistent with a curious hybrid idea, at least for the stimulus attribute of space: multisensory neurons can play one role in scaling spatial information in individual modalities (e.g., receptive fields do not change) in one dimension, and simultaneously in another dimension play a second role by integrating the inputs from these modalities to determine their overall effect on behavior.

These observations of the response properties of multisensory neurons raise interesting questions about the subjective consequences of activating them. For example, since intensity is represented in the central nervous system by a frequency code (i.e., in terms of the frequency of action potentials), might the intensity of stimuli in different modalities be judged along the same scale because they produce similar levels of activity in common multisensory neuronal pools throughout the brain? If so, multisensory neurons would play an integral role in cross-modal judgments. In this regard, it would be interesting to use the multisensory stimulation methods described in part IV to enhance or depress visually evoked response frequencies with nonvisual stimuli and determine how this affects judgments of visual intensity.

Andreassi and Greco noted in 1975 that the neural substrate for the visual-auditory interactions they were studying was not known. It is still not known. Nor are the substrates for the variety of intersensory interactions discussed above. The paucity of information about such fundamental questions illustrates the rudimentary stage at which the field is at this time. For while the perceptual phenomena demonstrate that interactions among different sensory modalities are commonplace and that constancies among the modalities must exist in order to use them together effectively, there is no comparable body of literature describing the neural mechanisms that underlie them. Nevertheless, there is a good deal of information about the location in the brain where inputs from different modalities converge. Presumably the approach we have adopted in studying the interactions among these inputs at the single neuron level (see part IV) will provide information applicable to these phenomena and some impetus to others to combine neural and perceptual studies in ways that will shed further light on their interdependence.

2 Sensory Convergence in Different Phyla

In the previous chapter, the "unity of the senses" concept was discussed with regard to sensory differentiation during early postnatal life. However, proponents of the concept have not restricted it to ontogeny. Rather, the concept extends to evolution as well, and its evolutionary component closely parallels its description of individual development. Briefly, the different sensory modalities are thought to have evolved from an undifferentiated and therefore "supramodal," primordial system, one that is not particularly selective about what it responds to. In such a system all effective sensory stimuli, regardless of whether they are chemical, thermal, mechanical, radiant, or of some other form, are thought to have had equivalent consequences based on their intensity: high-intensity stimuli evoked avoidance or withdrawal behaviors, and low-intensity stimuli evoked approach behaviors. The appearance of specialized receptors sensitive to only one form of environmental energy is thought to have reflected the evolutionary process of specialization and, hence, of sensory differentiation (von Hornbostel 1938; Bower 1974; Marks 1978; Butterworth 1981).

There is a certain "face," or apparent, validity to these ideas. Extant organisms that are considered primitive do withdraw from high-intensity mechanical, thermal, and radiant stimuli, and other specialized receptors do appear in more complex animals. However, there are also substantial differences between classes of stimuli (especially chemical) that fall under the general headings of attractants and repellants, and their classification is largely independent of stimulus intensity. Furthermore, there is presently no support for the idea that all forms of environmental energy to which primitive organisms are responsive are transduced in the same way by the same receptors. Thus, support for a single, nonspecific ancestral sensory receptor is lacking. On the other hand, it seems quite unlikely that the earliest cell, which formed the entire primordial organism, would not have been supramodal (see below).

UNICELLULAR ORGANISMS

The most primitive eukaryotic organisms are unicellular, and extant examples evolved from stem species that appeared about 1.4 billion years ago. The eukaryotes were derived from prokaryotes (the most ancient unicellular organisms—living bacteria are modern examples) in a marine environment. Unlike their prokaryotic antecedents, unicellular eukaryotic organisms developed a rich assortment of internal organelles (e.g., mitochondria, true cilia, mitotic spindles, nuclei). Extant species also lead much more diverse sensory lives than might be expected of beings dependent on only one cell to carry out all life functions. *Paramecium*, a very mobile ciliated protozoan, is one of the best-studied microbes. Although classified as a protist (just a cut above bacteria), it is often considered an "animal" by those who study its behavior and membrane properties.

Left to its own devices, a paramecium tends to swim about in a forward spiral. When confronted with mechanical, thermal, chemical, or photic stimuli, it changes its direction and/or speed of movement (Jennings 1906; Grell 1973). The ionic mechanisms by which it senses a mechanical stimulus and then reacts to it have been worked out by Naitoh, Eckert, and co-workers (Eckert et al. 1972; Naitoh and Eckert 1973; also see Kung et al. 1990).

Paramecium's membrane potential is normally negative, as are the membrane potentials of neurons in complex animals. But when forward movement causes the animal to bump into an object, the collision depolarizes the anterior membrane via an inward current of divalent cations. This depolarization, or receptor potential, is spread electrotonically into the cilia and triggers the opening of voltage-sensitive calcium channels, thereby initiating another potential: a regenerative, calcium-based action potential (although it is not a classic all-or-none type potential). The influx of calcium that takes place during this action potential causes the cilia to reverse the direction of their power stroke, and the animal now backs away from the object, as shown in figure 2.1. Very shortly thereafter, the potassium channels open, the calcium channels close, and the forward power stroke of the cilia is reinitiated. Just before forward movement resumes, the paramecium "tumbles" so that the forward movement is in a slightly different direction and it moves around the impediment. The opposite happens if the rear end of the animal is prodded: the mechanical stimulus initiates a hyperpolarizing receptor potential produced by the outflow of potassium ions due to a transitory increase in potassium conductance. This positive outward current accelerates the beating frequency of the forward-swimming power stroke of the cilia, and the animal accelerates forward and away from the prod (figure 2.1). In short, the cell membrane is nonhomogeneous: its anterior aspect (particularly its ventral surface) is specialized for the initiation of depolarization and the induction of backward movement, and

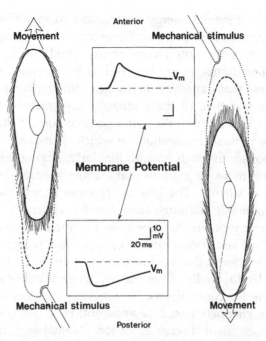

Anterior

Movement

Mechanical stimulus

V_m

Membrane Potential

10 mV
20 ms

V_m

Mechanical stimulus

Movement

Posterior

Figure 2.1 Effects of mechanical stimulation on *Paramecium*. Prodding the posterior of *Paramecium* (*left*) hyperpolarizes its membrane (V_m) and accelerates forward movement. In contrast, prodding its anterior (*right*) induces membrane depolarization, which reverses the stroke of the cilia, thereby driving the organism backward. (Modified from Ogura and Machemer 1980)

its caudal aspect (particularly its dorsal surface) is specialized for the initiation of hyperpolarization and the induction of forward movement (Ogura and Machemer 1980).

Touch- and stretch-induced receptor potentials are common among, and even predate, protozoa (Eckert 1965; Naitoh and Eckert 1969; Wood 1970; Kung et al. 1990; Morris 1990). Interestingly, the molecular mechanisms by which primitive membranes mediate the sensory functions of transduction and excitation bear fundamental similarities to those that are operative in all higher organisms: receptor potentials and action potentials caused by the concentration gradients of common ions and their movement through specific membrane channels (Kung and Saimi 1982; Hille 1984). Thus, the sophistication of their organizational characteristics often belies the term "primitive."

In modern unicellular organisms such as *Paramecium* there is already a good deal of channel specificity, and the ion channel by which the receptor potential is generated is distinct from that responsible for the action potential (de Peyer and Machemer 1978; Ogura and Machemer 1980). Furthermore, despite the fact that the sensory receptors that initiate these membrane changes to touch or chemical stimulation remain to be described (van Houten and Preston 1988), it is generally accepted that there is receptor specificity as well, and that different forms of environmental energy are transduced by different receptors. Certainly this is true in the case of protozoa with "eyespots." Thus, depolarizations of the anterior membrane produced by organic repellants and other chemicals are believed to be mediated by receptors other than those that transduce mechanical stimuli (Kung and Saimi 1982), despite the fact that all these stimuli may produce the same behavioral responses through the same sorts of current fluxes. For instance, there are protozoan mutations in which chemoreception is disrupted, but responses to touch remain. Similarly, among existing prokaryotic organisms there are mutants that are unresponsive to one or more attractants or repellants. The loss of response is not due to interference on the motor side (although such mutations also exist), but to a defect in transducer proteins that precludes the initial phase of stimulus transduction (Boyd and Simon 1982). Consequently, receptor and channel specificity characterize the most primitive organisms living today.

Undoubtedly, if the ancient progenitors of today's species were available for comparisons, evolutionary changes in sensory receptors and ion channels would be apparent; Hille (1989) should be referred to for an excellent discussion of ion channel evolution. There is no way to know the range of environmental stimuli to which these early receptors were sensitive, for even in the most complex species, receptors may have broad sensitivities or be sensitive to only a very narrow range of stimuli (Altner et al. 1983; Necker 1983). Some somatosensory receptors in the skin, for example, are broadly tuned and can respond to a variety of thermal and mechanical stimuli, other receptors, such as photoreceptors, are far more specialized and some are tuned to rather narrow wavelengths of light. Nevertheless (and despite the fact that much of the work on the evolution of channels and sensory receptors is, of course, speculative), it seems probable that the earliest unicellular animals had membranes with at least one mechanosensitive and numerous varieties of chemosensitive receptors.

While the observations presented above are not consistent with a primitive supramodal system at the receptor level, at the cellular level animals such as protozoa are supramodal by the very fact that they are one-celled beings responding to more than one sensory stimulus. In this context, and at this level of analysis, the "unity of the senses" is self-evident. The paramecium's behavior is a direct product of the synthesis of the stimuli to which its membrane is responsive—a multisensory integrator of the most elemental form. Direction of movement is not a choice, but, rather, depends on the sum of depolarizing and hyperpolarizing potentials induced by sensory inputs (regardless of their modality) on different membrane regions (a summation process not unlike the interaction of excitatory and inhibitory postsynaptic potentials derived from different sites of the neuronal membrane in mammals). Cellular differentiation and specialization were necessary to achieve sensory segregation and to progress from primitive obligatory multisensory summators like *Paramecium* to animals capable of regulating responses to sensory stimuli based on criteria other than their sign (i.e., attractant versus repellant) and relative intensity.

Evolutionary forces are apparent in macroscopic as well as microscopic anatomy, and just as the many extant ion channels evolved from far fewer progenitors (Hille 1984; Kung et al. 1990), many of the complex sensory organs that exist in multicellular animals were derived from fewer earlier forms. The eye, for example, is thought to have been derived from one sort of touch receptor (Gregory 1967; see Land and Fernald 1992 for an excellent discussion of the evolution of eyes), while the inner ear is thought to have evolved from another, probably hair cell mechanoreceptors, and not, as some had believed, from vestibular or lateral line organs (Northcutt 1986). As increasingly complex body forms evolved, there was a coincident increase in sensory specialization and segregation.

INVERTEBRATES

Primitive Species

The first step in the process of sensory segregation was the development of the simplest multicellular invertebrates. There are staggering numbers of invertebrate species alive today, and they vary widely in their ecological adaptations, their complexity of form, and their sensory processes. Very few invertebrates have been studied with respect to the questions addressed here, and disagreements concerning the capabilities of some of these animals are ongoing. Consequently, there are obvious hazards in generalizing across so broad and complex a group. Nevertheless, one can roughly categorize them into simpler and more complex forms, and clearly somewhere within invertebrate evolution there occurred the transition from multisensory animals to animals in which sensory segregation and multisensory integration could coexist.

Sponges, the lowest of the multicellular species, have no nerves or muscles. The animal consists of a loose network of cells (Mackie and Singla 1983), and the information derived from receptor activation on one part of the animal can have direct access to the cellular aggregate via protoplasmic continuity. Some form of stimulus identification takes place, since the animal ingests food and withdraws from harmful stimuli. However, this does not appear to require that inputs be segregated according to modality and directed to spatially segregated cellular populations. Similarly, in some primitive coelenterates, such as some species of medusae, sensory signals are transformed via conductive epithelia (Mackie and Passano 1968). The sensory signals are transmitted in all directions simultaneously, so that sensory segregation is also not possible. However, it is within this phylum that nerve cells, synapses, and nerve nets first appeared and cellular aggregates formed specialized sensory organs, such as those for detecting rotation and vibration of the body (statocysts) and photic (ocelli) stimuli. While the advent of specialized sensory organs sets the stage for sensory segregation, and these are obvious in coelenterates, as yet there is no evidence that it was actually achieved in these animals. Despite the presence of a primitive nervous system, there are no organized interneurons or ganglia in coelenterates, and much of the function of these early neurons may be secretory and hormonal in nature (De Ceccatty 1974). In most of the coelenterates that have been studied, impulses can pass readily among many cells, both neural and nonneural, via electrotonic coupling (De Ceccatty 1974; Anderson and Schwab 1982), so that different sensory stimuli may have access to large portions of the body and might indirectly render all cells in these regions multisensory. However, the difficulties in recording from the small cells in some coelenterates (e.g., anthozoans such as sea anemones and corals) slowed the pace of research in this phylum for some time. Although this situation changed with advanced technology and choices of preparations (Passano and McCullough 1962; Anderson and Mackie 1977; Anderson and Schwab 1982), conclusions about sensory segregation still must be tempered until more comprehensive evaluations of possible sensory selectivity are available.

The First Encephalized Species

An enormous leap in complexity and response flexibility occurred with the appearance of a more sophisticated, though still primitive, nervous system in the phylum Platyhelminthes (flatworms). The advent, elaboration, and fusion of ganglia produced an encephalized, bilaterally symmetrical animal with what can be considered a brain and a peripheral nervous system (i.e., plexus). The development of elongated axons, already beginning in coelenterates with the introduction of nerve rings and giant motor axons, becomes far more evident in platyhelminths and allows for the transmission of information over long distances without involving every intervening cell. In this way selective inputs and outputs can be maintained.

While it is anyone's guess which metazoan first developed truly unisensory afferents, it is likely to have been an early platyhelminth. Yet, even among modern platyhelminths that are available for study, the documentation is incomplete, and, to our knowledge, no one has conducted a systematic study in which all effective sensory stimuli for that animal are used in an effort to determine the selectivity of individual neurons. Nevertheless, the evidence for unisensory afferents in platyhelminths is strongly suggestive. Oddly enough, it comes from studies of bimodal cells.

Solon and Koopowitz (1982) found that there are bimodal neurons in the marine flatworm brain and that their responses to the offset of illumination and vibration can be habituated separately. Interestingly, only illumination offset could dishabituate the vibration response (even current injection into the cell could not), and vibration could not dishabituate the light offset response. The most parsimonious explanation of these findings is that there is modality segregation in peripheral afferents, so that these unimodal peripheral afferents can be habituated prior to their convergence on bimodal central interneurons. Indeed, habituation to vibration has been demonstrated in the peripheral plexus of decerebrate flatworms. Modality segregation may also exist in the animal's central nervous system, as some central interneurons already exhibit submodality segregation: separate vibration-sensitive and tactile-sensitive interneurons have been identified, and vibration sensitivity can be selectively blocked pharmacologically (Koopowitz 1975).

Advanced Invertebrates

Apparently, the capability for simultaneous segregation and integration among sensory modalities appeared quite early in the elaboration of nervous systems. By the time the more complex invertebrate species developed, the basic plan seen even in the most sophisticated vertebrates was already present: sensory inputs are transduced by elaborate, modality-specific organs, are then relayed to centralized structures over closely knit afferent pathways for further signal processing and evaluation, and, finally, signals are sent to the effector organs via well-defined output pathways. At this stage of evolution a mixture of unisensory and multisensory afferents is also apparent.

Invertebrates such as crustaceans (e.g., lobsters and crayfish), for example, have a multitude of large and small bristly hairs, or setae, on their walking legs (figure 2.2). These sensory organs contain modified ciliary cells that are bipolar, having their cell bodies in the periphery, with one end (the dendrite) projecting outward toward the tip of the hair and the other (the axon) projecting into the central nervous system, much like the processes of vertebrate first order olfactory and dorsal root neurons.

The setae contain receptors sensitive to chemical and mechanical stimuli and are quite effective in facilitating feeding. They are particularly sensitive to fish extract (Hatt and Bauer 1980), with individual afferents exhibiting remarkable sensitivity to amino acids, amines, or pyridines (Bauer and Hatt 1980). Presumably, the pattern of activity across the population of afferents is the signal the animal's brain uses to recognize the stimulus. The setae also are used to transduce mechanical stimuli (Tautz and Sandeman 1980), and a subpopulation of their peripheral afferents are bimodal. As such, these afferents provide a substrate at the most peripheral locus in the nervous system at which interactions among the simultaneous or sequential mechanical and chemical stimuli can occur during the acquisition of food. Hatt (1986) has shown that

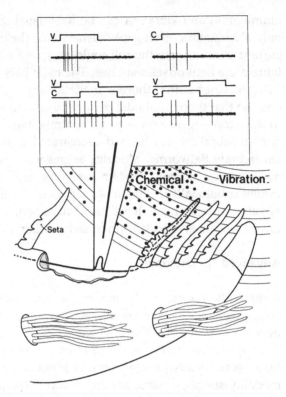

Figure 2.2 Multisensory integration in crayfish setae. The schematic at the bottom shows the opened exoskeleton of the walking leg of a crayfish. An axon innervating a seta is exposed, and a suction electrode has been applied to that axon to record action potentials (vertical spikes in oscillograms at top). The onset and offset of chemical (C) and vibratory (V) stimuli are indicated by the upward and downward deflections of the traces above the oscillograms. Note that when the vibratory stimulus precedes the chemical, more spikes are evoked than when these stimuli are presented individually. When the sequence is reversed, the chemical stimulus inhibits responses to the vibratory stimulus. (Responses were drawn from descriptions of Hatt and Bauer 1980, figure modified from Hatt and Bauer 1980)

presenting a vibration just before a chemical stimulus lowers the activation thresholds and enhances the responses of these peripheral afferents (figure 2.2). One would expect a summated response of this sort to enhance the detection of food, and indeed, coupling tactile and chemical stimuli facilitates feeding in another marine invertebrate, *Aplysia* (Rosen et al. 1982). However, reversing the stimulus sequence, so that the chemical stimulus occurs first, reduced the afferents' responsiveness to vibration (figure 2.2). The adaptive significance of this inhibitory interaction is not immediately apparent.

The selective pressures on afferents to segregate sensory inputs must have been very different from the pressures on the central interneuron and output branches of the nervous system. The progress in afferent selectivity becomes obvious with the development of dedicated peripheral sensory organs (e.g., eyes, ears, noses) whose inputs to the nervous system are carried by unisensory afferents. The same afferent segregation that allowed some areas of the brain to be devoted to modality-specific processing enabled other areas to pool sensory inputs and become specialized for the synthesis of information across two or more modalities. Synthesizing multisensory information in central neurons is a particularly effective way for responses to be enhanced when individual cues are weak. It may also facilitate the identification of an external event, especially when individual cues are ambiguous. Multisensory convergence on output pathways is an efficient way to produce the identical behavioral response no matter which sensory channel signals its need. This distinction between afferent selectivity and central and efferent sensory integration is an organizational pattern characteristic of all mammals, and the essence of the scheme is already apparent in complex invertebrates. The escape systems in crayfish are good examples.

While multisensory integration occurs in some crayfish peripheral afferents, its sensory systems have evolved to the extent that only a comparatively small afferent population deals with both chemical and mechanical cues. Similarly, visual, tactile, and proprioceptive inputs converge at various levels of its neuraxis, but the percentage of neurons that are multisensory increases from afferent, to higher order central, to descending limbs of the nervous system (Wiersma and Mill 1965; Tautz 1987). Thus, in the presence of a good deal of afferent selectivity, the "decisions" and descending signals that mediate the animal's behavior generally represent a synthesis of sensory inputs. This is evident in its so-called voluntary escape behaviors. These escape behaviors are mediated by nongiant efferent fibers in the nerve cord, which have long latencies, variable responses, and react to a host of threatening gestures transduced by visual, tactile, and vibratory receptors. The crayfish's response is simply to swim away from the threat. At the same time, the animal maintains a more reflexive and less multisensory system for immediate escape responses to stimuli that touch the body or are rapidly approaching it. These stereotyped "tail flip" responses, which are not a normal component of swimming behavior, occur within milliseconds of the stimulus and are mediated by giant fibers in the nerve cord (Wiersma 1947; Wine and Krasne 1972). Similar systems with varying degrees of multisensory convergence are found in worms (Krasne 1965), cockroaches (Dagan and Parnas 1970; Ritzmann et al. 1991), and other invertebrate animals. This contrasts with mammals, in which all sensory stimuli can evoke all varieties of escape behavior.

Insects

The tendency for modality-specific afferents to converge on central and efferent neurons is a general characteristic of complex invertebrates, regardless of their specific ecological niche (see Horn 1983), and while the integration of these inputs has not been widely investigated, important information has been generated in insects. For these animals the integration of information from highly developed peripheral and internal sensory organs is essential to control flight (Strausfeld et al. 1984; Hensler 1989; Olberg and Willis 1990; Maronde 1991).

In a series of recent studies reminiscent of multisensory studies in mammals (see part IV), the critical interplay among the different sensory signals has been evaluated in individual insect interneurons. For example, male gypsy moths, like other male insects (and the males of more "advanced" species), are impelled by sex pheromones to locate the female. Visual cues, as well as the pheromone concentration in the air, are used to determine and maintain the male's flight course. Motoneurons controlling this flight have their dendrites in the thoracic ganglion, where they can be contacted by a class of efferent interneurons that descend from the brain via the ventral nerve cord (Willis and Carde 1990). Intracellular recordings have shown that a substantial proportion of these descending interneurons are multisensory (Olberg and Willis 1990), and that they are able to integrate cues from different modalities to alter their response profiles and, thus, their influence on flight motoneurons. In some cases, neurons that are unresponsive to either a pheromone or a visual stimulus become responsive to their combination. In others, the visual response becomes selective to a particular direction of movement when a pheromone is present, while in still other neurons (which already exhibit direction selectivity) direction selectivity is markedly enhanced by a pheromone (figure 2.3). The effects are not unidirectional, and the visual stimulus can also affect the response to the pheromone (figure 2.3).

Presumably, direction selective visual responses are important because they enable the male moth to use cues from the ground and forest canopy to maintain his flight course to the female while avoiding any obstacles along the way. An optomotor system of this sort also seems well suited for continual correction of the misdirections that could occur from the moth's curious zigzag flight pattern. However, since female insects also fly, and males occasionally have goals other than females, nonpheromone influences on moth flight are also necessary.

If the moth is like other insects, once aloft, the problems inherent in maintaining a set course with shifting winds, changing visual cues, and the overcorrections in steering that characterize insect flight can also be solved by integrating proprioceptive, tactile (i.e., wind against the antennae and body parts), and visual cues. The integrators that pool the signals from these external and internal receptors have been labeled "descending deviation detectors" by some investigators. They are a class of efferent interneurons in the nerve cord that project to the animal's flight-controlling and body-controlling thoracic motoneurons and are the equivalent of the descending interneurons in the moth discussed above. Their multisensory properties have been studied most closely

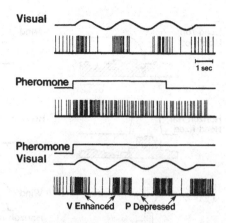

Figure 2.3 Multisensory integration in a moth interneuron. This neuron responded to a moving visual stimulus (V, *top*) and to a pheromone (P, *middle*). The oscillogram at the top illustrates that the movement of a visual stimulus in one direction elicited more impulses than movement in the other. The pheromone elicited a long train of impulses. However, when the two stimuli were combined, the neuron's directional tuning was enhanced significantly and the long discharge train of the pheromone was no longer apparent. (Modified from Olberg and Willis 1990)

in locusts (Rowell and Reichert 1986; Hensler 1989), although similar mechanisms appear to be operative in other flying insects (Strausfeld and Bassemir 1985; also see Horn 1983).

Many of the descending deviation detector neurons are particularly responsive to the visual cues induced by changes in the position of the horizon. They fall into different groups, depending on whether they are sensitive to horizon shifts in one direction or the other and, because they are also influenced by vestibular cues, whether the horizon shift is induced by roll, yaw, or pitch during flight. But most of these neurons behave in similar fashion: they are direction selective, and the greater the change in the position of the horizon, the bigger the change (increase or decrease) in their phasic neural activity. By balancing the activity of these different neurons, the animal maintains an orientation normal to the horizon. The responses to visual signals are quite sensitive to inputs from proprioceptors in the head and neck, as well as to wind against the body. Examples of the integration of these inputs are provided in figure 2.4. In the first, the visual response was enhanced by the presence of a coincident proprioceptive signal, even though proprioception alone was inadequate to affect the neuron. In the second, the neuron required multisensory cues (visual and wind) to provide any useful signal of the animal's orientation. Individually, the cues were not helpful at all. These multisensory interactions appear to be the invertebrate equivalents of the multisensory interactions in mammals that will be discussed in subsequent chapters, and suggest that the mechanisms for multisensory integration in higher organisms were laid down quite early in evolution. ·

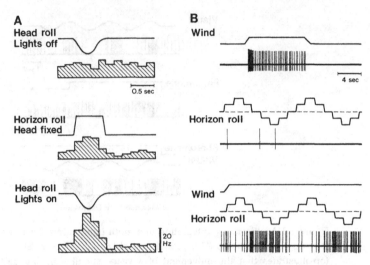

Figure 2.4 Visual-proprioceptive and visual-tactile interactions in a locust interneuron. (A) At the top, the effect of stimulating neck proprioceptors by head roll in the dark is illustrated in a peristimulus time histogram of impulses. Note the absence of an obvious response. In the middle, a response to a visual stimulus is elicited by horizon roll when the head is fixed. At the bottom, a significant response enhancement is shown to the combined proprioceptive/visual stimulus (head roll in the light) (B) The activity of another neuron is recorded in response to a tactile stimulus induced by wind (*top*), a visual stimulus induced by horizon roll in the light (*middle*), and a combined tactile-visual stimulus (*bottom*). The neuron became sensitive to one direction of visual movement in the presence of the tactile stimulus, and the tactile response was dramatically reduced during the opposite direction of visual movement. (Modified from Hensler 1989)

Invertebrate Associative Learning

The pooling of multiple sensory cues in the same neurons also provides a mechanism for substituting one cue for another, as in the cross-modal phenomena discussed in the previous chapter. Through the formation of cross-modal associations, an organism can learn to organize anticipatory responses to sequential stimuli of different modalities. Although it seems to be a higher order function, cross-modal association can already be effected in invertebrates via multisensory neurons. This is evident from the studies of associative learning in the marine snail, *Hermissenda crassicornis*. Alkon and co-workers (Alkon 1983) have shown that visual, vibratory, and chemosensory inputs converge at several sites along the afferent and efferent pathways of this animal. They were able to use a conditioning paradigm to transfer the normal behavioral response to water turbulence (i.e., vibration) to a light stimulus. Presumably, various response transferences could have been effected with different stimulus combinations.

Hermissenda protects itself from water turbulence by attaching its "foot" to a hard surface in deeper and calmer water. Because it feeds on surface-dwelling microorganisms called hydroids, it has a natural propensity to move toward light. By repeatedly presenting a light stimulus about 1 sec before a rotatory stimulus that mimicked water turbulence, the investigators were able to suppress the animal's normal tendency to react to light by approaching it. After multiple pairings of the light and rotation, the light stimulus alone caused the animal to react as if it were in turbulent water: it attached itself, or remained attached, to the hard surface of the water-filled glass tube in which training took place. The association could last for weeks. Fortunately, *Hermissenda* can survive for weeks without feeding, and repeated presentations of the light in the absence of rotation led to extinction of the learned response. By tracing the pathways by which light-induced and turbulence-induced behaviors are effected, and evaluating the molecular changes that took place during conditioning, these investigators were able to show that conditioning depends on altering the ionic changes induced by light and rotation in a class of cells sensitive to both stimuli.

One usually thinks of associative phenomena as requiring a far more elaborate nervous system than *Hermissenda* has, perhaps because the examples of associative learning and anticipatory responding to which we are usually exposed are those that have been described in mammals. Undoubtedly, the best known is that of Pavlov's dog, and in this example of Pavlovian or classical conditioning, repeatedly presenting a sound and then placing food on a dog's tongue led it to salivate in response to the sound alone (Pavlov 1927). Almost as well known is Skinner's instrumental conditioning paradigm, in which a neutral sensory stimulus (e.g., a light) cues a rat (or other mammal) to behave in a certain way to obtain food (Skinner 1938). Successful conditioning depends on the animal making an association between the neutral stimulus and the taste of the food. Yet, the work in *Hermissenda* indicates that the neural bases for cross-modal association were established in comparatively simple organisms. It would be interesting to compare the mechanisms of cross-modal conditioning in different phyla to determine how closely the fundamental mechanisms parallel one another. Although conditioning at the level of the single neuron has been studied in the vertebrate nervous system for some time, the specific roles that multisensory neurons might play in this phenomenon, and the ionic mechanisms crucial to effecting it, have not been worked out. Examining these questions at each level of the mammalian nervous system seems like a Herculean task. Yet, the broad interest in the mechanisms of learning makes it quite likely that the necessary combinations of **in vivo** and **in vitro** studies are already ongoing somewhere.

VERTEBRATES

Afferent segregation by sensory modality reaches its peak in vertebrates. Yet, even here, there are instances in which multisensory integration takes place among first and second order afferent neurons. As noted in the previous discussion of perception in higher mammals, this is particularly true in the vestibular system, and the involvement of somatosensory and visual inputs on vestibular processing is a general vertebrate characteristic that is as evident in fish and amphibians (Dichgans et al. 1973; Hartmann and Klinke 1980; Caston and Bricout-Berthout 1984, 1985) as it is in mammals (Keller and Daniels 1975; Waespe and Henn 1979; Precht and Strata 1980; Cazin et al. 1980; Horn et al. 1983). Similarly, the lateral line system of teleosts, used for detecting water movement against the body, is influenced by descending visual signals (Tricas and Highstein 1990).

Discussions of the central locations of modality-specific versus multisensory neurons are easiest in mammals. It is here that the most information is available, and the mammal will be targeted in the discussion below. Yet despite the wide variations in the brains among and between mammalian and nonmammalian species, and a good deal of lively discussion about how these patterns may have evolved (Jerison 1973; Kruger and Stein 1973; Northcutt 1984; Glezer et al. 1988; Stein 1988b; Kaas 1989), it appears likely that the general trends of modality segregation and combination are applicable across vertebrate groups.

Among the many thousands of studies of primary sensory areas are some isolated reports of nonsomatosensory influences on cortical (and second order) somatosensory neurons (Jabbur et al. 1971; Atweh et al. 1974; Zarzeki et al. 1983), nonauditory influences on neurons in auditory cortex (Sams et al. 1991), and nonvisual influences on thalamic and visual cortical neurons (Morrell 1972; Fishman and Michael 1973; Spinelli et al. 1968; Buisseret and Maffei 1983; Chalupa et al. 1975). Despite these studies, it is generally accepted that (unlike the vestibular system) visual, auditory, and somatosensory stimuli initiate a stream of modality-specific information along their primary projection pathways. It is, perhaps, best to moderate the current dogma somewhat and accept the likelihood that there are circumstances in which some modulation by other sensory inputs can take place even along these projection systems, and this will be implicit when primary projection systems are referred to below as modality-specific. However, the dramatic difference between the relative purity of the sensory signals along the primary projection pathways and the high incidence of multisensory convergence outside them warrants retention of the distinction. An example of a primary sensory pathway is the somatosensory projection, in which peripheral afferents from the skin project to the dorsal column nuclei, which send their projections to their dedicated thalamic relay nucleus (the ventrobasal complex), which, in turn, projects to the primary somatosensory cortex (SI).

The parcelling of sensory projections produces a sensory duality in the central nervous system that is evident at the level of the brain stem and above: modality-specific primary projection pathways coexist with other projection systems in which various sensory inputs converge and interact with one another. And there are a myriad of multisensory convergence sites, the most intensively studied of which is the superior colliculus (and its nonmammalian homologue, the optic tectum), a structure in the midbrain involved in attentive and orientation behaviors. The sensory convergence patterns, multisensory integration and literature relevant to the superior colliculus are considered extensively in much of the remainder of this book and will not be dealt with in detail in this chapter. However, this structure is only one of many sites in the central nervous system at which multiple sensory inputs come together on the same neurons.

Multisensory neurons are also well represented throughout the reticular activating system, from the lower brain stem to the midbrain (Amassian and Devito 1954; Bell et al. 1964; Yen and Blum 1984). One of the roles played by the reticular formation is that of general arousal, and it is able to influence the activity of widespread target nuclei through its dense network of connections. It makes intuitive sense that an activating system pools together information from different externoreceptors, since arousal responses must be evoked by all pertinent external stimuli regardless of the modality used to sense them. This pooling of sensory inputs in the reticular formation often takes the form of convergence on the same neurons, and is an example of conservative biology. But convergence is not limited to reticular areas of the brain stem, and multisensory integration is not limited to general arousal. Multisensory properties characterize structures with widespread as well as those with local projections, those involved in general modulation of nervous system activity, and those involved in more specific information processing regarding stimulus identification or localization.

At the brain stem level, multisensory neurons are found not only in reticular structures, but in the locus coeruleus (Grant et al. 1988), the external nucleus of the inferior colliculus (Itaya and Van Hoesen 1982; Tawil et al. 1983; Tokunaga et al. 1984), and the superior colliculus. At the thalamic level, the duality of modality-specific versus multisensory structures becomes more obvious. Nuclei within the primary projection pathways, such as the lateral geniculate (visual), medial geniculate (auditory), and ventrobasal complex (somatosensory), which preserve modality-specific signals, coexist with structures in the posterior and lateral thalamus (Hotta and Terashima 1965; Wespic 1966; Avanzini et al. 1977; Chalupa and Fish 1978; Rasmussen et al. 1984), in which multisensory convergence is common. Because primary and nonprimary thalamic nuclei have different patterns of projections to cortex, it is no surprise that this duality is retained at this next level, where polysensory cortices abut areas devoted specifically to one modality or another. A similar situation appears to exist in elasmobranchs (Ebbesson 1980; Bodznick 1991) and suggests that this is characteristic of many complex vertebrates.

Cortical regions can receive afferents that are already multisensory, as well as converging inputs from different unisensory thalamic nuclei (Jones and Powell 1970). The primate superior temporal and intraparietal cortices are well endowed with multisensory neurons (Benevento et al. 1977; Bruce et al. 1981; Hikosaka et al. 1988; Mistlin and Perrett 1990; Duhamel et al. 1991; Watanabe and Iwai 1991; Stein et al. 1993), as is its frontal and prefrontal cortex (Rizzolatti et al. 1981a,b; Ito 1982; Vaadia et al. 1986). A similar situation exists in cat, with multisensory convergence present in parietal (Dubner and Rutledge 1964; Toldi et al. 1984; Stein et al. 1993), frontal (Clemo and Stein 1983), and orbital (Fallon and Benevento 1977; Benevento et al. 1977; but see Hicks et al. 1988) cortices. Polysensory cortical areas are generally considered "association" areas, and while much needs to be learned about their specific functional capabilities, they are believed to play essential roles in higher perceptual, cognitive, and attentive behaviors. Obviously, the integration of multisensory information is important for these processes and for the emotional and learning processes that may accompany them and there is good reason to believe there is extensive multisensory convergence in cingulate cortex, the parahippocampal gyrus, and hippocampal areas, which function in concert with polysensory association cortex (Van Hoesen 1982; Room and Groenewegen 1986; Isaacson 1987; Musil and Olson 1988; West and Michael 1990).

On the output, or premotor/motor limb of the central nervous system, multisensory neurons also abound. The basal ganglia is an interrelated group of structures playing an essential role in coordinating movement, and visual, auditory, somatosensory and noxious stimuli can influence single neurons here in various combinations (Barasi 1979; Schneider et al. 1982; Wilson et al. 1983; Hikosaka and Wurtz 1983; Strecker et al. 1985; Hikosaka et al. 1989). A similar situation exists in the outputs of the superior colliculus (see part IV), and various regions of the cerebellum (Freeman 1970; Caan et al. 1976; Barasi 1979; Waespe and Henn 1981; Chapman et al. 1986; Graf et al. 1988; Archer et al. 1990; Azizi and Woodward 1990).

There can be little doubt that multisensory integration can play a significant role in just about every kind of behavior. While we are concerned primarily with mammals in this volume, it should be obvious from the preceding discussion that multisensory convergence and integration per se are present in comparatively simple organisms, and are likely to be ancient schemes that characterized even the primordial animal. It is segregation among existing modalities and the creation of new ones that occurred during the evolutionary process.

It seems logical (albeit a bit teleological) that during the process of developing differentiated sensory systems, mechanisms were preserved or elaborated for using their combined action to provide information that would be unavailable from their individual operation. That this process is dependent upon some coherence in stimulus features is evident in the heightened perceptual awareness induced by related (i.e., spatially and temporally coincident) combinations of sensory stimuli, as well as in the perceptual and behavioral anomalies evident when unrelated, or spatially conflicting, stimuli are combined (see chapter 1). It is this coherence to which we will return in subsequent chapters in an attempt to outline what we know of the rules of multisensory integration at the level of the single neuron. In this context it would have been particularly interesting to know the course by which multisensory interactions were changed from the presumably linear systems operative in unicellular organisms such as *Paramecium*, to the nonlinear systems that characterize more complex animals. Unfortunately, such information is not available.

II   Multiple Sensory Systems and the Superior Colliculus

The superior colliculus is impressive in the multiplicity of sensory modalities represented within it and in the widespread areas of the nervous system that it affects directly through the activity of its output neurons. These features reflect its broad impact on sensory and motor functions and will be dealt with extensively here. But before discussing its different functions, it is essential to review what is known about the organization of the structure, where it gets its different sensory and motor inputs from, and where it sends its outputs to effect behavior. These anatomical features are reviewed briefly in chapter 3 and help put into context the information we have about how its multisensory properties facilitate its role in overt behavior. A more complete description of afferent-efferent relationships and the internal structure of the superior colliculus can be found in Huerta and Harting (1984a,b).

In discussing the functions of the superior colliculus in chapters 3–5 it will become evident that more is known about its visual role and the visual properties of its neurons than about any other modality represented within it. Thus, in chapters 3 and 4, which deal with superior colliculus organization and some historical perspectives about its function, more space is devoted to the visual modality than to the auditory and somatosensory modalities. Nevertheless, the receptive field features of each of the sensory modalities represented in the superior colliculus serve to screen the information that has access to its circuitry, and, ultimately, to its integrative mechanisms. A good deal of information is now becoming available about how superior colliculus neurons deal with nonvisual (i.e., somatosensory, auditory, and noxious) as well as visual stimuli; these data are reviewed in chapter 5.

As a general guide, the roles of all modalities represented in the superior colliculus center about attentive and orientation behavior, such as that illustrated in the schematic shown in figure II.1. Therefore, the combinations of different sensory inputs are evaluated here within an attentive-orientation context. However, ideas about the roles of the superior colliculus and its relationship with higher centers in the brain have changed considerably over time, and many of these conceptual changes are also discussed.

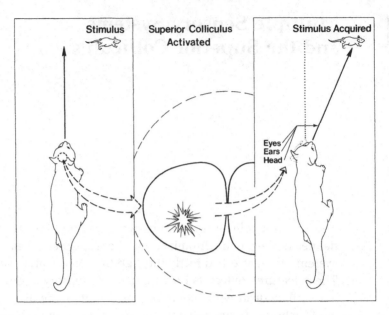

Figure II.1 Behavioral role of the superior colliculus. A sensory stimulus activates a localized region of the superior colliculus which, in turn, directs the eyes, ears, and head toward that stimulus.

The details regarding the multisensory properties of deep-layer superior colliculus neurons have been documented most extensively in the cat; therefore, although they have been found to be generalizable to other species, the discussions here will deal in far greater depth with deep-layer neurons in cat. In some contexts, however, the inclusion of data from the more superficial layers or other species is illuminating and will be included. But if nothing is said about which animal is being discussed or which division of the structure is at issue, it is safe to assume the data come from the deep layers of the cat superior colliculus.

3 Anatomical Organization of the Superior Colliculus

LAMINAR PATTERN

The term *colliculus* derives from the Latin word for hill, *collis*. After blunt dissection of the brain to remove the caudal aspect of the cerebral cortex, the superior colliculi do indeed appear as a pair of large symmetrical bumps forming the dorsal surface of the midbrain (figure 3.1). In nonmammalian vertebrates this tissue forms an actual roof over a large ventricle, hence the name *optic tectum* (tectum is the Latin word for roof). Some investigators tend to ignore this distinction and refer to the superior colliculus as the *tectum* (although purists cringe at this, and we will avoid that usage here). It may seem odd, however, that the converse is not also true. No one refers to the optic tectum as the colliculus, and nearly everyone labels inputs to the superior colliculus as something-tectal (e.g., retinotectal, corticotectal) and outputs from it as tectal-something (e.g., tectoreticular, tectospinal). There is simply no accounting for the biases in nomenclature.

From top to bottom, the superior colliculus is composed of seven alternating cellular and fibrous layers (Kanaseki and Sprague 1974) (figure 3.1), but the structure is usually divided operationally into only two parts: superficial (layers I–III) and deep (layers IV–VII). However, this distinction is not at all obvious when one inspects a section through the tissue: there is no space, no large blood vessel, nor any dramatic cytoarchitectural boundary to separate the upper three from the lower four layers. Rather, it is a convenient operational division based on overall differences in neuronal morphology, afferent-efferent projections, physiological properties, and behavioral involvements (see Edwards 1980; Stein 1984a for further discussion).

While commonalities exist among the superficial and deep divisions (e.g., both contain visually responsive neurons arranged visuotopically), it is the deeper and not the superficial layers that receive inputs from different sensory modalities and from motor-related structures as well. It is also the deeper layers that send their outputs to areas of the brain stem and spinal cord that are most directly involved in positioning the peripheral sensory organs and are thus strategically involved in the

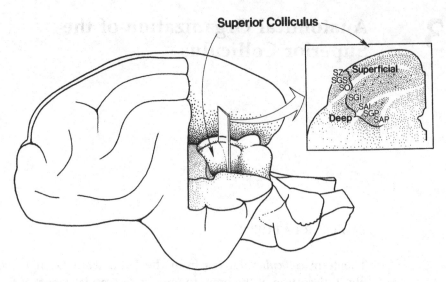

Figure 3.1 Location and laminar pattern of the cat superior colliculus. In this schematic of the cat brain, the posterior region of the cerebral cortex is removed to reveal the superior colliculus in the midbrain. A coronal section (*upper right*) shows its laminar organization. Superficial layers include: SZ, stratum zonale; SGS, stratum griseum superficiale; SO, stratum opticum. Deep layers include: SGI, stratum griseum intermediale; SAI, stratum album intermediale; SGP, stratum griseum profundum; SAP, stratum album profundum.

transformation of incoming sensory information into motor commands. Consequently, the multisensory attentive and orientation functions of the superior colliculus involve its deeper layers; if the superficial layers play any role in these behaviors it is an indirect one.

AFFERENTS

Two general characteristics of deep layer afferents are readily apparent: (1) they converge on the superior colliculus from a large number of morphologically and functionally diverse structures (table 3.1), and (2) in cross section many of them appear to be distributed in discontinuous "patches" across the mediolateral extent of the tissue. Actually, each patch is more like the face of a slice through a horizontally oriented tube, so that it runs for some distance rostrocaudally through the structure. These horizontal tubes of tissue are comparatively well confined within a dorsoventral tier thereby giving the region a patch and matrix appearance. The arrangement seems well suited to parceling information within the structure, and has given rise to the concept of a functional mosaic here (Huerta and Harting 1984a). This idea of an internal mosaic is consistent with other anatomical observations, including those indicating that inputs arise primarily from modality-specific regions of the brain (figure 3.2) and their terminal territories may be partially segregated from each other. However, a functional correlate of the patchy anatomical mosaic has not yet been established.

Table 3.1 Afferents to Deep Laminae of the Cat Superior Colliculus

Ascending	Descending
Visual	
Retina	Posterior and lateral suprasylvian
Pretectum	cortex
Ventral lateral geniculate n.	Anterior ectosylvian sulcus
	Orbital cortex
Somatosensory	
Sensory trigeminal complex	SIV (anterior ectosylvian sulcus)
Dorsal column n.	Para SIV (anterior ectosylvian sulcus)
Lateral cervical n.	Rostral lateral suprasylvian cortex
Spinal cord, dorsal horn	
Auditory	
Exterior n. inferior colliculus	Field AES (anterior ectosylvian
N. brachium inferior colliculus	sulcus)
N. sagulum	
Dorsomedial periolivary n.	
N. trapezoid body	
Motor	
Substantia nigra	Frontal eye fields
Entopeduncular n.	
Medial, interposed, and lateral n. of	
deep cerebellum	
Perihypoglossal n.	
Zona incerta	

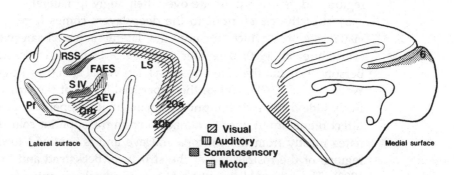

Figure 3.2 Cortical projections to deep superior colliculus of the cat. Corticotectal neurons are most heavily concentrated in the extraprimary cortical areas, including LS (lateral suprasylvian sulcus); areas 20a and 20b; AEV (anterior ectosylvian visual area); SIV (fourth somatosensory area); FAES (auditory field in the anterior ectosylvian sulcus); Orb (orbital gyrus); RSS (ventral bank of the rostral suprasylvian sulcus), Pf (prefrontal, presylvian sulcus) and, on the medial surface of the hemisphere, area 6 (cruciate sulcus).

Sensory Afferents

Sensory afferents converge on superior colliculus neurons from ascending (e.g., retina, spinal cord, brain stem) and descending (cerebral cortex) sources. The descending component of this system is quite robust and has been demonstrated repeatedly. Yet even in the absence of this documentation, one would have assumed that such projections existed, for there is no reason to assume that higher order functions are coded in the ascending afferents to the superior colliculus, or that they are organized within intrinsic superior colliculus neurons themselves; it is intuitively obvious that such influences must be present to ensure that experience and environmental circumstances dictate which stimuli have the most potent effect on the attentive and orientation circuitry of this structure. The most likely source of this sort of context- and experience-based control system is the neocortex, and the normal impact of cortical influences on superior colliculus neurons becomes quite evident when cortex is removed: the excitability of superior colliculus neurons is immediately depressed and many of their response properties are altered.

The degree to which superior colliculus neurons depend on cortical inputs varies among modalities. Visual responses are far more depressed by cortical deactivation than are somatosensory, and somatosensory responses are more depressed than are auditory. Nevertheless, regardless of modality, each of the descending corticotectal sensory projections follows the same pattern: it originates from an extraprimary region and its projections are overwhelmingly ipsilateral.

Most of the *visual* input to the deep layers comes from extrastriate visual regions, which include the lateral suprasylvian visual area (Tortelly et al. 1980; Baleydier et al. 1983; Segal and Beckstead 1984; Berson 1985) and the anterior ectosylvian visual area (Mucke et al. 1982; Wallace et al. 1991). Unlike the superficial layers of the structure, relatively little direct retinal input terminates in its deeper layers. Whatever direct retinal input does terminate deep in the superior colliculus originates mostly from the contralateral eye and is confined to the upper regions of the rostral half of the structure (Beckstead and Frankfurter 1983). The limited distribution of retinocollicular inputs confines their effect to a minority (Berson and McIlwain 1982; Mize 1983a,b) of superior colliculus neurons, and the number of such inputs is sparse. Other structures that also send comparatively sparse visual inputs to deep layers include the ventral lateral geniculate nucleus and the pretectum (Edwards et al. 1974, 1979; Huerta and Harting 1984b). These observations, coupled with the minimum influence of superficial influences on deep-layer neurons (see below), explain why the visual responses in the deep superior colliculus depend so heavily on descending influences from cortex.

Despite the widely held view that superficial and deep superior colliculus function as independent entities, a number of recent reports have shown that some fibers from the superficial visual layers project to the deep layers in hamster (Rhoades et al. 1989; Mooney et al. 1988), cat (Behan and Appell 1992), and monkey (Moschovakis et al. 1988a). Furthermore, some deep-layer neurons extend their dendrites into superficial layers in cat (Moschovakis and Karabelas 1985). These anatomical observations suggest that some communication occurs between the two divisions of the structure. Recently, Mooney and co-workers (1990) confirmed this by showing that visual influences from superficial layers contribute to the responsiveness of deep layer neurons in hamster. Similar observations have not yet been made in any other species. In fact, depressing the activity of superficial layer neurons in cat by deactivating their cortical inputs has no obvious influence on the functional integrity of deep layer neurons (Ogasawara et al. 1984; Stein 1988a). Nevertheless, it is hardly likely that the connections that exist between superficial and deep layers in cat and monkey are nonfunctional—their function simply has not yet been demonstrated.

The *somatosensory* corticotectal projections arise principally from the dorsal bank of the anterior ectosylvian sulcus (Stein et al. 1983; McHaffie et al. 1988), an extraprimary somatosensory area that had generally been considered an "association" area, and therefore an area that was not expected to have separate, well-organized (i.e., maplike) sensory representations.

The discovery in the early 1980s that a portion of the anterior ectosylvian cortex had a well-organized somatosensory representation was the result of several attempts to demonstrate corticotectal projections from a variety of somatosensory cortices. Even the most sensitive axonal tracing techniques failed to show such projections from any of the three cortical areas (SI–SIII) known at the time to be somatosensory. Because it was difficult to believe that the neocortex made no somatosensory contribution to the superior colliculus, studies using retrograde tracing techniques were then undertaken to reexamine this issue. The retrograde experiments demonstrated a heavy corticotectal projection from a largely unexplored area of cortex, the anterior ectosylvian sulcal cortex. Subsequent studies showed that these corticotectal projections terminated in the superior colliculus in a way that seemed to parallel the distribution of somatosensory neurons there (Stein et al. 1983). Finally, recordings from anterior ectosylvian neurons demonstrated that they were somatosensory and were organized into a well-formed map of the body (Clemo and Stein 1982; see also Burton et al. 1982). The region was designated SIV, because it is the fourth cortical area in cat shown to have a map of the body surface (Clemo and Stein 1982). Another extraprimary somatosensory area, the rostral lateral suprasylvian sulcus, in which a fifth somatosensory map appears to exist (Clemo and Stein 1984; Mori et al. 1991), also projects to the superior colliculus (Stein et al. 1983).

These studies on the anterior ectosylvian sulcus demonstrated the existence of a heretofore unknown somatotopically organized cortex, and also showed that this area is a principal corticotectal region. However, the data also made it seem misleading to continue designating the anterior ectosylvian area as an "association" area of cortex. Combining the results of several studies shows that there are three separate sensory representations along the curve of the anterior ectosylvian sulcus: SIV dorsal and rostral; a visual area called AEV somewhat ventral and caudal to SIV (Mucke et al. 1982; Olson and Graybiel 1987); and an auditory area, Field AES (Clarey and Irvine 1986; Meredith and Clemo 1989), at the caudal extreme. These regions are separated from one another by border zones, where unimodal neurons from different modalities and multisensory neurons are intermingled (Clemo et al. 1991).

There is also an ascending component contributing to the somatosensory representation in the superior colliculus, and, unlike the modest retinotectal projection to deep layers, it is quite heavy. Somatosensory projections originate from the contralateral sensory trigeminal complex, dorsal column nuclei, lateral cervical nucleus, and spinal cord (Edwards et al. 1979; Huerta and Harting 1984b; Blomqvist et al. 1978).

The *auditory* corticotectal projection to the superior colliculus comes only from the Field AES region of the anterior ectosylvian sulcus (Meredith and Clemo 1989). However, the ascending component of the auditory representation arises from a variety of sources (primarily contralateral), including the brachium of the inferior colliculus, the external nucleus of the inferior colliculus, the nucleus sagulum, the dorsomedial periolivary nucleus, and a region medial to the trapezoid body (Edwards et al. 1979). As in the somatosensory representation, these ascending inputs are much heavier than the ascending component of the visual representation.

Motor Afferents

Motor afferents arise from numerous (primarily ipsilateral) sources as well. Perhaps the best known direct motor corticotectal projection is the one that comes from the frontal eye fields in cat and primate (Sprague 1963; Astruc 1971; Kunzle and Akert 1977; Kawamura and Konno 1979; Leichnetz et al. 1981) and from the motor cortices in rodents (Leonard 1969; Beckstead 1979; Neafsey et al. 1986; Leichnetz et al. 1987; Sesack et al. 1989). In addition, heavy inputs from the basal ganglia, via substantia nigra pars reticulata, contact the majority of superior colliculus output neurons (Moschovakis and Karabelas 1985) and play a critical role in the oculomotor (and other) behaviors they subserve (Hikosaka and Wurtz 1983; Chevalier and Deniau 1987). Other oculomotor-related inputs are also derived from the zona incerta, thalamic reticular nucleus, and nucleus of the posterior commissure. Afferents also arrive from the deep nuclei of the cerebellum, including the medial and posterior interposed nuclei, and from the related perihypoglossal nucleus (Edwards et al. 1979; Kawamura et al. 1982; May et al. 1990).

Other afferents, whose functions are not well understood, originate from the contralateral superior colliculus, locus ceruleus, raphe dorsalis, parabrachial nuclei, reticular formation, and hypothalamus (Edwards et al. 1979). Some of these latter inputs may play a role in varying the likelihood of a given movement depending on the prior experience and immediate needs of the organism.

MORPHOLOGY OF NEURONS

Superior colliculus neurons have various shapes, and range in size from 8 to 60 μm in diameter (Norita 1980); their morphology and neurochemistry have been reviewed recently by Grantyn (1988). The somatic and dendritic surfaces of the larger of these neurons are covered extensively (up to 83%; Behan et al. 1988) with synaptic terminals, of which eight different types have been identified (Norita 1980). The dendritic arborization is almost always broad, and in many instances can span 1.2–1.4 mm (Moschovakis and Karabelas 1985); therefore, it is not unusual for a neuron's dendritic tree to cross the borders of adjacent layers, or even to spread from the deep division of the structure into the superficial layers (Mooney et al. 1984; Moschovakis and Karabelas 1985; Moschovakis et al. 1988a). Because of the extreme variations among somatic and dendritic properties, axonal distribution has become a critical factor in establishing morphological patterns or groupings. Neurons whose axons arborize and remain within the superior colliculus are few, and these interneurons appear to represent only a minor proportion of the population (at least in primate; see Ma et al. 1990). In contrast, neurons with efferent projections predominate and, according to their projection patterns, fall into one of four categories (figure 3.3). The targets of these different output pathways are described below.

EFFERENTS

Deep-layer efferent projections reach their target structures via four output pathways: one that ascends to thalamus (ascending), one that projects to the opposite superior colliculus (commissural), and two that descend to brain stem and spinal cord (one crossed and one uncrossed descending output pathway). These are shown schematically in figure 3.3. Presumably, the ascending outputs alert higher centers to changes in the functional conditions of deep-layer neurons; the commissural projections coordinate the activity of the two superior colliculi and may play a role in vergence movements of the eyes in response to approaching targets (Edwards 1977; Edwards and Henkel 1978); the descending efferents are involved in initiating behavioral responses to stimuli by repositioning the eyes, head, limbs, and—in species that can

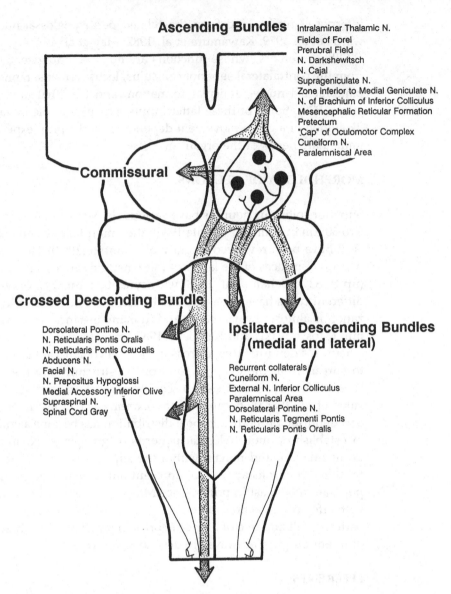

Ascending Bundles

Intralaminar Thalamic N.
Fields of Forel
Prerubral Field
N. Darkshewitsch
N. Cajal
Suprageniculate N.
Zone inferior to Medial Geniculate N.
N. of Brachium of Inferior Colliculus
Mesencephalic Reticular Formation
Pretectum
"Cap" of Oculomotor Complex
Cuneiform N.
Paralemniscal Area

Commissural

Crossed Descending Bundle

Dorsolateral Pontine N.
N. Reticularis Pontis Oralis
N. Reticularis Pontis Caudalis
Abducens N.
Facial N.
N. Prepositus Hypoglossi
Medial Accessory Inferior Olive
Supraspinal N.
Spinal Cord Gray

**Ipsilateral Descending Bundles
(medial and lateral)**

Recurrent collaterals
Cuneiform N.
External N. Inferior Colliculus
Paralemniscal Area
Dorsolateral Pontine N.
N. Reticularis Tegmenti Pontis
N. Reticularis Pontis Oralis

Figure 3.3 Efferent targets of deep superior colliculus. Axons of deep-layer neurons exit the superior colliculus via one or more of the four major efferent paths: ascending, commissural, crossed-descending (also called the predorsal bundle or tecto-reticulo-spinal tract), and ipsilateral descending (with medial and lateral components). (The targets of these tracts were identified by Grantyn and Grantyn 1982; Huerta and Harting 1984b; Moschovakis and Karabelas 1985; and Vidal et al. 1988.)

move them—the ears and whiskers (Martin 1969; Kawamura et al. 1974; Graham 1977; Edwards and Henkel 1978; Kawamura and Hashikawa 1978; Coulter et al. 1979; Weber et al. 1979; Holcombe and Hall 1981; Grantyn and Grantyn 1982; Huerta and Harting 1984b; Dean et al. 1986).

Because most descending output neurons are the sites of extensive multisensory convergence, each of the sensory representations has access to at least some of the same efferent, or premotor, circuitry. This enables the different sensory systems to initiate the same behaviors via some of the same neurons. The different output circuits summarized in figure 3.3 all play roles in the production of overt behavior; it is not yet clear what the various sensory convergence patterns are in each of these circuits. Some neurons that project in the crossed descending bundle reach only as far as the pontine tegmentum, while others in the same bundle project to the spinal cord (Keay et al. 1990; Redgrave et al. 1990; Olivier et al. 1991; May and Porter 1992). While there is extensive divergence within this system (Grantyn and Grantyn 1982), all outputs do not go to all the target structures of the superior colliculus.

Although information about sensory convergence patterns among output neurons is incomplete, there appear to be different patterns of modality convergence on the different subclasses of output neurons, at least in rats. Their tectospinal neurons are heavily influenced by somatosensory stimuli (Rhoades and DellaCroce 1980; Chevalier et al. 1984; Westby et al. 1990; Keay et al. 1990), while those projecting to the contralateral pontine reticular formation are activated preferentially by auditory stimuli (Keay et al. 1990). Presumably, similar differences in efferent projections are present in other species, although their purpose is not yet known. In cats, most of the descending efferent neurons are known to be multisensory, but a significant proportion of unimodal neurons is also represented in this population (Meredith and Stein, 1985). At the moment there is no reason to believe that unimodal efferent neurons are dedicated to controlling only one set of peripheral sensory organs, and the advantage of modality specificity, or a specific multisensory convergence pattern on a specific output neuron, remains unclear. We will return to this issue when dealing with the parallels among the sensory modalities represented in the deep layers (chapter 6).

4 The Superior Colliculus and Vision: Some Historical Perspectives

VISUOMOTOR INVOLVEMENT

For most of the history of interest in the superior colliculus, its functional role was thought to be restricted to the visual system and to relate solely to the generation of eye movements. Only comparatively recently has the structure become a significant focus for investigators interested in the sensory aspects of vision, and even more recent is its inclusion in studies of audition and somatosensation. Previously, the sensory components of vision, audition and somatosensation were believed to be the province of the primary thalamocortical systems, and the recognition of the superior colliculus as a multisensory structure playing a pivotal role in transforming different sensory signals into orientation behaviors has been late in coming.

Yet, despite the initial attention to only one aspect of superior colliculus function and the relatively crude technology available to early investigators, some of the observations they made proved to be remarkably astute. Even a cursory examination of this early literature makes one realize how far back seminal ideas in the field can be traced and how much greater a role insight played in their generation when scientific technology was less sophisticated. The eye movement organization of the superior colliculus, a topic still under active investigation, was first demonstrated using rather gross electrical stimulation techniques more than one hundred years ago (Adamuk 1870). Stimulation of the anteromedial aspects of the structure evoked contralateral, upward, and parallel conjugate deviations of both eyes, while lateral stimulation elicited conjugate, contralateral, and downward excursions. This early concept of a movement map has been confirmed repeatedly and extended to include movements of the head and, in some species, the external ears, whiskers, and even the body. In brief, the activation of neurons in a localized region of the structure produces shifts of the eyes, ears, and head to focus on the location in space that is represented at the stimulation site.

One would predict from these early observations that under normal circumstances the activity of neurons at any given site should discharge in a way that codes for the execution of only a very specific movement, and that the specified movement should shift systematically at different sites so that the entire range of orientation movements is represented. The demonstration that this is, indeed, the case had to await the development of techniques that allowed investigators to record from individual neurons in behaving animals; these observations will be dealt with below in the section entitled Modern Concepts of Visuomotor Function. For now, however, it is essential only to keep in mind that the "motor" circuitry of the superior colliculus has a maplike organization.

Questions soon arose about the cues that might be used during early ontogeny to construct a motor map in the superior colliculus. One early postulate was that the motor organization is guided by sensory inputs, a suggestion derived from Apter, who also described the organization of retinal inputs to the superior colliculus in 1945. She demonstrated that strychnine crystals applied to different sites on the superior colliculus could evoke eye movements that turned the eye toward the area of visual space represented at the stimulation site (Apter 1946). This sensory-motor registry was confirmed in subsequent studies and led to the hypothesis that both the sensory and motor representations are organized in retinal coordinates. The presumptive purpose of this registry was to produce a "visual grasp reflex," or "foveation" response, that would bring the eye to bear on the stimulus that initiated the movement. Despite its tantalizing simplicity and face validity, the retinal coordinate hypothesis could not account for later observations that the retinal map exceeds the range of possible eye movements (the map of visual space is described in detail in chapter 6), that ballistic eye movements (i.e., saccades) can be made to nonvisual targets, which of course have no retinal coordinates, and that some saccades evoked from the rear of the superior colliculus produce eye movements that directly violate a retinal coordinate system in order to reach a specific position in the orbit (Roucoux and Crommelinck 1976; Guitton et al. 1980; McIlwain 1986).

The inadequacy of the hypothesis is perhaps best illustrated by a particularly clever experiment demonstrating that displacing the eye from its intended trajectory during a saccade (by electrically stimulating the brain during the eye movement) does not interfere with it reaching its appropriate destination (Sparks and Mays 1983); it simply corrects for the disruption and the radically altered retinal coordinates. How does it do this?

One possibility is that disrupting retinal coordinates is of little significance because the neurons use a "motor error" signal based on the relative locations of the eye in the orbit and the target. These kinds of observations resulted in the hypothesis that the overall organization of the superior colliculus is based on motor rather than sensory coordinates. In this view the sensory map follows the motor coordinate system, and presumably does so developmentally as well. This suggestion is consistent with the observation that spatially "correct" eye movements can be evoked electrically from subregions of the superior colliculus during the first few days of postnatal life, long before visual activity can be elicited in the structure (Stein et al. 1980). It also helps to explain a variety of functional properties of the structure. However, there is no current theory that adequately details the mechanisms by which motor organizations can guide the development of sensory maps here, or which explains the observation that one sensory representation (i.e., visual) exerts a critical developmental influence on the formation of another's (i.e., auditory) map (King et al. 1988; Withington-Wray et al. 1990a; Knudsen and Brainard 1991). Perhaps an initial, gross topographical guidance system serves to get most of the machinery of the sensory and motor representations roughly in place. This could be followed by more subtle, dynamic, use-dependent mechanisms in which both sensory and motor inputs fine-tune the alignments of their own maps based on the consequences of their coordinated use. The issues of map construction will be dealt with in more detail in chapters 6, 8, and 12.

Modern Concepts of Visuomotor Function

The advent of the alert, behaving paradigm was a boon to understanding the properties of movement-related neurons in the superior colliculus. The first of such studies, in the 1970s in monkeys and cats (Straschill and Hoffmann 1970; Wurtz and Goldberg 1971; Robinson and Jarvis 1974; Sparks 1975, 1978; Crommelinck and Roucoux 1976; Straschill and Schick 1977), dealt mainly with eye movements and showed that many superior colliculus neurons exhibit a burst of activity that is time-locked to the onset of the saccadic eye movement made when shifting visual attention from one location to another, as we do when reading. These "premotor" neurons were activated before movements in a particular direction and of a particular amplitude; in other words, these neurons have "movement fields" much like the receptive fields of sensory neurons (figure 4.1). Neurons with similar movement fields are located in the same region of the superior colliculus, and different movement fields are represented systematically across the structure much like sensory receptive fields. Their presence and distribution account for the eye movement map that had been demonstrated with cruder electrical stimulation techniques.

These premotor neurons are not simply involved in the initiation of an eye movement, but are involved in determining its speed, direction, and amplitude as well. Once the presaccadic bursts of these neurons exceed a certain threshold discharge frequency, a saccade is evoked (Grantyn and Berthoz 1985), and the frequency of their discharge trains determines the velocity of the eye movement (Berthoz et al. 1986; Munoz and Guitton 1986). In addition, there is another type of neuron whose activity is vital to controlling the eye during its excursion. Called

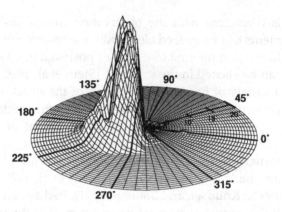

Figure 4.1 Movement field of a saccade-related burst neuron. This neuron was active before eye movements that were 0–14° in amplitude and directed from 190–315° in angle. This area of movement space in which the neuron is active is termed its movement field. (From D. Sparks, unpublished data)

"motor error" neurons, they generate a low-frequency, long-duration discharge that continues as long as there is a difference between current eye position and the target (Mays and Sparks 1980; Munoz and Guitton 1985; Jay and Sparks 1987a; Munoz et al. 1991a,b). Since there is no proprioceptive feedback from extraocular muscle receptors to directly signal current eye position to superior colliculus neurons (Nelson et al. 1989), it is thought that this signal is provided by a corollary discharge (Guthrie et al. 1983) from extrinsic neurons (see chapter 7).

Saccadic eye movements are expressed not only in response to visual stimuli, they can be elicited just as easily by nonvisual, remembered, or even imagined stimuli. So it is not surprising to find that premotor superior colliculus neurons will exhibit characteristic high frequency bursts prior to saccades evoked by visual, nonvisual, and even by remembered (Jay and Sparks 1984; Sparks 1989) or predicted (Munoz and Guitton 1989; Munoz et al. 1991b) targets.

The oculomotor range of the cat is rather limited—estimated to be no more than about 25 degrees from a fixation point directly ahead (Crommelinck and Roucoux 1976; Evinger and Fuchs 1978; Collewijn 1977), even when maximal movements are evoked by direct electrical stimulation of the superior colliculus (Stein et al. 1976a). In normal behavior, cats rarely, if ever, make such large eye movements, which seems to create a bit of a problem. Because the animal's visual field extends 90–105 degrees temporal (Sprague 1966a; Sherman 1974a,b; Hardy and Stein 1988), it is far broader than its oculomotor range. So when far peripheral targets appear, the eye movements they initiate will not have the range required to acquire the target. Primates have a somewhat larger maximum oculomotor range than cats, but they still have the same problem. The simplest solution to this difficulty turns out to be the one that has been selected: peripheral stimuli activate neurons in caudal superior colliculus and these neurons initiate programs that move the eyes and head in concert. These "gaze shifts" appear to have a control mechanism similar to that for eye movements alone. Thus, perturbing an ongoing gaze shift by brain stimulation results in a "correction" so that the proper target is still acquired (Pelisson et al. 1989), just as is the case for the perturbed eye movement described earlier. Apparently the gaze shifts are coded in body-centered coordinates.

These "gaze shifts" have formed the basis of an intriguing model involving the superior colliculus. Munoz and Guitton (1989, 1991) and Munoz and co-workers (1991a,b) identified two functionally distinct classes of output neurons that project to contralateral gaze-control centers. One type is located in an area far rostral in the structure that corresponds to the part of the visuomotor map representing the area centralis. These neurons are tonically active when the animal fixates a target. However, during gaze shifts their activity ceases and, at the same time, the second neuronal type becomes active. These gaze shift neurons are represented at all other sites in the structure, and their burst activity produces an eye movement or a coordinated eye and head movement to center the target. The position of the active population of neurons within the visuomotor map of the superior colliculus determines the amplitude and direction of the shift in gaze.

It might appear, then, that activation of a limited number of neurons at a single location in the superior colliculus would evoke a well-directed eye or eye and head movement. Certainly this is true. However, it does not appear to be the way the system normally works. That is, an eye movement normally is not initiated by the activation of only those neurons that have the same, or even very closely related, movement fields. Every movement initiated by this circuit involves a host of active neurons, spread over a surprisingly large area of the superior colliculus, many of which have significantly different movement vectors (see McIlwain 1991 for a more comprehensive discussion). The movement produced is the average of the vectors of the population of neurons recruited (Van Gisbergen et al. 1987; Lee et al. 1988; Munoz and Guitton 1991; Munoz et al. 1991a,b). So, for example, if a movement is directed 10 degrees left along the horizontal meridian, neurons in the right superior colliculus with vectors on, below, and above the horizontal meridian will be recruited simultaneously. If the cooperation of neurons with movement vectors below the horizontal meridian are eliminated because they are damaged or anesthetized, the averaged vector will change and the movement will shift, and will now be to a point above the horizontal meridian (Lee et al. 1988). According to the Munoz and Guitton (1989) model, in the acquisition of this or any other target, there is a moving locus of activity in the superior colliculus that continues to drive the movement to the target. For example, a gaze shift to a stimulus in the far left visual field consists of a sequential activation of successive subregions of the right superior colliculus from caudal to rostral (Munoz et al. 1991a; also see chapter 5) corresponding to decreasing levels of motor error as the eyes become progressively nearer to the target. However, it is not yet clear how this model incorporates the movement fields of premotor neurons.

SENSORIMOTOR TRANSFORMATION

There is a certain artificiality in separating neurons into sensory and motor categories. It is easier to discuss them this way, but it gives the impression that most superior colliculus neurons perform only one very specific function when quite the opposite is true. As will be become evident here, many superior colliculus neurons have multiple sensory and motor properties and are involved in a variety of different circuits and functions. From a design standpoint, this makes maximal use of a limited population of neurons, but from an analysis standpoint it makes it difficult to fit them into neat, exclusive categories.

A good example of the multiple roles of a single neuron is the neuron with saccade- or gaze-related activity. Many of them also respond to sensory stimuli, and their movement fields and visual receptive fields are in register (Mohler and Wurtz 1976). This may make it seem as if the task of transforming the visual cue into the motor program that directs gaze toward the cue is quite straightforward. Unfortunately for those who seek to understand this system, it is not. The spatial coordinates of the sensory signals (e.g., retinal) initiated by the cue are quite different from the coordinates of the motor signal that must be initiated in order to turn to look at it (e.g., the contraction and relaxation of many extraocular and neck muscles must be coordinated and must take into account their current and desired position). Thus, the nervous system usually makes a clear distinction between the signals related to sensory and motor activity, even in the same neurons. These signals differ not only in frequency, pattern, and duration, but in timing as well. Furthermore, the sensory evoked activity can end many milliseconds before the beginning of the premotor discharge that ultimately produces the saccadic eye movement (figure 4.2; Mohler and Wurtz 1976; Mays and Sparks 1980; Jay and Sparks 1987a; Munoz and Guitton 1991).

What is most surprising in the behavior of these neurons is the absence of a tight temporal coupling between the responses to the sensory stimulus that initiates the oculomotor process and the premotor discharges that actually drive the movement. Consider for a moment the following example. An animal is trained to make an eye movement every time a light comes on in its peripheral visual field. The light is always effective in driving superior colliculus neurons, and thus, a particular saccade-related neuron that we are interested in for this example (its visual receptive field overlaps the light) responds to light onset with 100% reliability. The sequence is always: (1) light on, (2) sensory

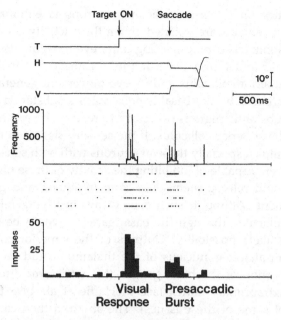

Figure 4.2 Sensory and premotor signals from the same neuron. This neuron showed a burst of impulses in response to visual target onset (upward deflection of the uppermost electronic trace, labeled T), as well as just before a saccadic eye movement that contained horizontal (H, second trace) and vertical (V, third trace) components. The two bursts of neuronal activity are displayed in an instantaneous frequency histogram and a raster display just below it (each dot = one neural impulse, and each of the five rows of impulses is the response to a single trial). A peri-event time histogram at the bottom summarizes the data by summing the discharges contained in each raster. (From Jay and Sparks 1987a)

response, (3) premotor discharge, and finally (4) eye movement. The premotor discharges of this neuron will always begin at a set period of time before the eye movement, but the interval between its sensory responses and the premotor discharge (and thus, the eye movement) is quite variable, as if they were unrelated to each other (Mohler and Wurtz 1976; Jay and Sparks 1987a; also see the example provided in figure 12.2). Moreover, many other premotor neurons involved in generating this eye movement will not even exhibit sensory responses to the light onset. These observations raise a disturbing question: Why have a sensory response on a neuron that exhibits premotor activity when that sensory response appears unrelated to the movement? No ready answer is available, and efforts are being made to determine where the sensory signal goes before being converted into the eye movement command.

A likely component of the circuit that might help explain what happens to the sensory signal before it initiates a premotor discharge is the basal ganglia. Most efferent neurons of the superior colliculus that could be involved in eye movements receive inputs from the substantia nigra (Karabelas and Moschovakis 1985), the output structure of the basal ganglia. When these nigrotectal neurons are silenced so that their influence on superior colliculus neurons is eliminated, irrepressible eye movements are initiated; when their activity is enhanced or their action is mimicked pharmacologically, eye movements are suppressed (Hikosaka and Wurtz 1985). It appears, then, that the efferent output of the superior colliculus and its eye movement generation function are held in check by the basal ganglia via the substantia nigra. Turning off the substantia nigra is necessary to release the eye movement generator in the superior colliculus. If the sensory signals in the deep superior colliculus (especially those in neurons with both sensory and motor activity) were capable of inhibiting the activity of these nigrotectal neurons, they could release themselves from inhibition and generate an eye movement. Although such a pathway, involving relays from the superior colliculus through the basal ganglia, would be polysynaptic, it seems a likely possibility. Outputs of the superior colliculus that go to the intralaminar nucleus of the thalamus could be relayed to a receiving portion of the basal ganglia (i.e., striatum) directly and indirectly via extraprimary cortex (see McHaffie et al. 1993 for a recent discussion of some of these issues). The striatum then can inhibit the inhibitory influences of the nigrotectal projection, allowing for the buildup of the high frequency discharge in superior colliculus neurons (the movement generator) that precedes a shift in gaze. The various links in this pathway can also account for the time difference between the sensory-evoked activity in the superior colliculus and the premotor discharge. It takes an appreciable length of time to relay through thalamus, cortex, and then the successive levels of the basal ganglia. Whether this indirect circuit can also account for the absence of a tight temporal coupling between the sensory and premotor components is not clear at this time.

Because a variety of movements can be evoked by electrical stimulation of the superior colliculus, it would seem reasonable to postulate that the same premotor neuron can code for more than one type of movement. Indeed, some of the descending efferents through which motor responses are initiated (e.g., tecto-reticulo-spinal neurons) in cats have extensive collateralizations within the brain stem to contact centers controlling both eye movements and head movements (Grantyn and Grantyn 1982). However, the mechanics underlying these functions indicate that a more complex plan might be required. Eye muscles require a much higher frequency of stimulation (often a factor of 10; Meredith and Goldberg 1986) for efficient contraction than those controlling the position of the head and ears (Stein and Meredith 1991). Therefore, the signals sufficient for eye muscles seem likely to overdrive others, and those sufficient for ears and neck would seem to be inadequate to drive the eye muscles. While there may be several plausible mechanisms to compensate for this mismatch, it is not clear at this point what the actual output plan is. On the one hand, there is evidence of at least some segregation among output neurons in terms of the sensory stimuli that activate them (some discharge only to a somatosensory or a visual stimulus, whereas others respond to targets of any sensory modality) and some segregation in the targets to which they project (Westby et al. 1990; Keay et al. 1990; Olivier et al. 1991; Redgrave et al. 1986; May and Porter 1992; also see Efferents, above). On the other hand, the extensive collateralization of other efferents suggests that either the same signals can somehow be used by different target structures, or that there is some change in the nature of the signals or their effects when they reach the various terminal arbors. This is an issue to which we will return when discussing multisensory convergence (see chapters 8 and 9).

Despite conceptual changes in the presumptive mechanisms by which superior colliculus neurons code appropriate gaze shifts, the fundamental hypothesis that there is a sensory-motor loop involving the superior colliculus remains intact: sensory activation of this structure results in the activation of a motor program that shifts the peripheral sensory organs to target the initiating stimulus. Currently, researchers are concerned not only with how the discharges of superior colliculus neurons generate these movements, but also with how the activity of superior colliculus neurons codes sensory stimuli and how this sensory activity relates to the initiation of the movements in the first place. Concepts of sensory coding in superior colliculus neurons are of particular importance in the present context, and they, too, have been radically altered over time, as much by changes in the social climate in which science is conducted as by the accumulation of empirical data.

SENSORY INVOLVEMENT

Changing Views of Visual Coding

Early assessments of both the sensory and motor roles of the superior colliculus were greatly influenced by popular evolutionary views. One of these, sometimes called "progressive encephalization of function," holds that during the transition from premammalian to mammalian forms over 180 million years ago, many of the functions of structures like the optic tectum (the premammalian homologue of the superior colliculus, and a structure which was once thought to underlie all the important visual functions in nonmammalian vertebrates) were taken over by the emergent neocortex. This required a tremendous elaboration of the sensory projections from thalamus to cortex to deliver the massive amounts of information that this new cortex would need to perform its functions. The geniculostriate system is a good example of a "recently" elaborated pathway from thalamus to cortex. Some who favor this view believe that the organizational differences among the central visual pathways of such extant mammals as dolphin, hedgehog, cat, tree shrew, and various species of monkey represent different stages in the elaboration and differentiation of the superior colliculus and visuocortical systems (Diamond 1967; Diamond and Hall 1969; Glezer et al. 1988).

Consistent with the notion that newer, or higher, centers took over the roles of lower, or older, structures is the observation that visual cortex lesions produce considerably greater visual defects in man than in other primates, and greater defects in monkeys than in cats, and so on down some presumptive phyletic line of brain complexity, whereas, conversely, optic tectum and superior colliculus lesions generally produce less severe defects as one goes up the same line.

Recent reevaluations of phyletic relationships question many of the assumptions of evolutionary lineage implied in this sequence (e.g., it is unlikely that cats are in a direct line to man) and, as will be discussed below, there is reason to question the assumption that specific functional roles were simply transferred intact from the optic tectum to the cortex. Yet, whether or not one can document a linear trend of increasing brain complexity along a given phyletic line, there seems little doubt that the brains and the behavioral repertoires of primates generally are more complex than those of carnivores, that those of carnivores generally are more complex than those of rodents, and so on. Undoubtedly, there are examples to the contrary, but in general, increasingly complex organisms exhibit progressively greater neocortical elaboration. It is more than likely that the latter determines the forms. A more highly elaborated neocortex is one that will be more involved in the decisions that release and coordinate overt behaviors and perhaps control many of their features, even if many of the behaviors are organized in subcortical centers. This is less an upward transference of function (Weiskrantz 1961) than a different way of sharing functional responsibilities among interrelated structures. The specific pattern with which different cortical and subcortical regions share functions in different animals no doubt depends on the ecological situations in which they developed and the neural processes that became available to them.

The various views and observations on the evolution of the brain led to two research strategies for understanding how the brain deals with visual information: one sought answers by using the so-called simpler systems of nonmammalian species as a model to understand basic principles by which the biological "hardware" works, and another sought answers in advanced mammalian models that were thought to be more directly comparable to man. The combination of ease of access to the optic tectum and Herrick's (1948) view of it as the supreme center of coordinating motor responses to sensory stimuli encouraged a great many investigators to favor the first strategy and use the optic tectum as a model. On the other hand, the view that the neocortex is the "highest" visual area in mammals, coupled with early clinical observations that lesions of primary visual cortex (i.e., striate cortex) rendered humans blind, led many others to become enamored of the second strategy and to use the geniculostriate system as a model.

Both strategies have been successful and a great deal of information has been generated about tectal function in fish, amphibians, reptiles, and birds, and about geniculostriate function in rodents, carnivores, and nonhuman primates. However, the very focused nature of these efforts resulted in somewhat restricted functional views, and in the effort to understand how these systems work, the roles of other visual areas received considerably less attention. Tectal researchers apparently had little impetus to examine either the functional properties of neurons in targets of ascending tectal efferents or the roles of the nonmammalian analogue (and possibly the homologue) of the geniculostriate system, the visual thalamo-telencephalic system. Similarly, researchers studying mammalian systems spent far less time on investigations of structures that were grouped together as "extrageniculostriate," a rubric that reflects the presumptive preeminence of the geniculostriate system in the formidable job of coding sensory input. Extrastriate cortex was thought to play a major role in using its inputs from striate cortex for abstract visual functions, and the superior colliculus was thought to provide the supportive reflex function of moving the eyes to the target of interest.

Modern Concepts

Recent studies have questioned some of the generalizations that resulted from many early experiments. For example, lesions of the optic tectum in some fishes do not produce the predicted blindness (Springer et al. 1977; Graeber 1984), whereas lesions of the supposedly less important telencephalon in these species produce deficits in pattern discrimination like those induced by cortical lesions in mammals. Similarly, telencephalic lesions in amphibians (i.e., frogs) produce sensory and attentive defects like those seen after cortical lesions in mammals (Traub and Elepfandt 1990). These observations certainly were not in keeping with earlier concepts of visual organization in nonmammalian species, nor were they consistent with the concepts of reorganization and functional segregation that were thought to take place during the evolutionary transition to early mammals.

Two Visual Systems

An abrupt fracture in the established concepts of superior colliculus function occurred after it was found that removal of a superior colliculus in the cat or hamster produced a dramatic neglect of contralateral visual stimuli despite an intact geniculocortical system (Sprague and Meikle 1965; Schneider 1967, 1969). This would not have been predicted given the idea that the role of the superior colliculus was limited to moving the eyes. Similarly, demonstrations that there are many representations of the visual field in mammalian neocortex (Woolsey 1981; Rosenquist 1985); that these extrastriate neocortical areas subserve some of the functions previously believed to be performed by striate cortex; and that the most encephalized species of all, man, exhibits some visual perceptions in the absence of striate cortex (Poppell et al. 1973; Weiskrantz et al. 1974; Zihl 1980; but also see Campion et al. 1983; Gazzaniga 1988) have led to a reevaluation of the prevailing dogma about how visual processes are organized in the mammalian brain and how this organization may have changed during the radiation and evolution of mammals. The observation that frogs with tectal lesions retain the capacity to discriminate stationary objects and that this discrimination depends on higher centers such as those in caudal thalamus (Ingle 1973b) suggests that mammalian evolution has elaborated on a substrate already laid down in amphibians. Attempts to examine possible anatomical and functional correlates between mammalian cortex and its presumptive homologue in nonmammalian species, the dorsal ventricular ridge, is only one example of a new awareness of the need for a more thorough comparison of functional homologies.

Sprague and Meikle's (1965) experiments with cats and Schneider's (1967, 1969) experiments with hamsters were of considerable importance in initiating modern concepts of superior colliculus function and promoting the upsurge of interest in this structure that began in the late 1960s. In the Sprague and Meikle experiments, cats with lesions of one superior colliculus exhibited a profound neglect of visual stimuli on the opposite, or contralateral, side (figure 4.3). The nature of the stimulus was largely irrelevant—threatening gestures and food were ignored equally; yet the animals were perfectly capable of turning to the contralateral side and moving in that direction without apparent motor impairment. Furthermore, they were entirely capable of navigating around

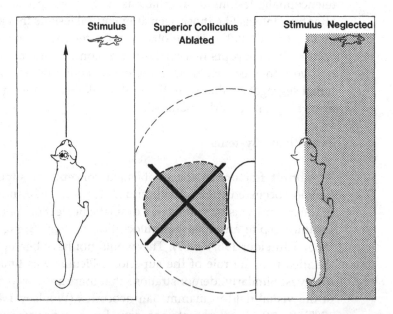

Figure 4.3 Superior colliculus ablation. A unilateral superior colliculus lesion produces contralateral sensory (visual, auditory, and somatosensory) deficits. The visual neglect is illustrated here.

obstacles on either side of them. The defect appeared to be one of integrating sensory and motor information. The term *visual neglect* was particularly appropriate in describing the behavior of these animals, who were not "blind" in the normal sense of the word. Soon thereafter, Schneider (1967) used circumscribed lesions to compare the visuomotor functions of the visual cortex and the superior colliculus in hamsters. He, too, noted that removal of a superior colliculus produced a neglect of contralateral visual stimuli, whereas visual cortex lesions produced difficulties in discriminating among visual patterns. Together these observations ushered in the concept of *two visual systems*, one primarily to subserve the analysis of stimulus detail, such as its pattern (the geniculocortical system) and the second to subserve visual attention and orientation behaviors (the superior colliculus).

The idea that there were two visual systems, entirely segregated from one another, one for "where" and another for "what," was a popular exaggeration of the implications of these studies. These two neural systems are linked anatomically and functionally, so that cortical lesions disrupt superior colliculus function and superior colliculus lesions inhibit eye movements and thus the scanning and learning of new patterns (see below). Nevertheless, the *idea* that this sort of extreme segregation of function existed in the visual system was provocative, stimulating substantial interest among visual scientists. Subsequent studies in many laboratories confirmed the observation that destroying the superior colliculus produced attentive and orientation defects of varying severity in different species (Casagrande et al. 1972; Goodale and Murison 1975; Albano et al. 1982; Dean and Redgrave 1984; Midgley et al. 1988). Curiously, however, lesions of just the superficial layers of the structure (where visual neurons are most densely represented) had no apparent effect on visual attentive and orientation behaviors (Casagrande et al. 1972). It was only when the deeper layers were involved that visual neglect became apparent. This result, coupled with morphological and physiological differences in superficial- and deep-layer neurons, was an important factor in the conceptual segregation of the superior colliculus into superficial and deep divisions, as discussed earlier.

It seems ironic that while the density and ease of studying superficial-layer visual neurons led to a disproportionate degree of attention being devoted to their properties, their behavioral role remains far more obscure than that of less frequently studied deeper-layer neurons. Nevertheless, it was the assumption that the dense visually innervated superficial layers were involved in attentive and orientation behaviors that provided the impetus for a host of physiological studies of neuronal properties in the superior colliculus. As an offshoot of this interest, the visual properties and, ultimately, the multisensory character of deeper-layer neurons were described as well.

Receptive Field Properties of Visual Neurons

Initial interest in detailing the properties of visually activated superior colliculus neurons centered on two basic questions: Which stimuli are capable of activating these neurons, and how do their visual receptive field properties differ from those in the geniculostriate system? Answering the first question was critical in determining which environmental stimuli have the greatest access to the circuitry of the superior colliculus; answering the second was important in formulating hypotheses about how the different physiological properties of cortex and midbrain might be tied to their different behavioral roles.

From the late 1960s through the early 1980s a great many physiological studies were conducted. Even though a variety of different species and methods were used in these investigations, the results showed good agreement among investigators on the fundamental properties of these neurons, and remarkable consistency across species as well. Although each neuron does not necessarily exhibit each of the following characteristics, these properties are commonly represented.

1. Their receptive fields are not divided into separate "on" and "off" zones as are those that characterize retinal and lateral geniculate neurons. Rather, they appear to be homogeneously organized.

2. Receptive fields are generally large compared to those in the geniculostriate system.

3. The receptive field is bordered by an inhibitory or "suppressive" zone. Consequently, when this zone is stimulated the response to the stimulus presented within the excitatory zone is degraded or suppressed.

4. The most effective stimulus is far smaller than the diameter of the receptive field.

5. Stimuli moved across the receptive field are far more effective than are stimuli that remain stationary and are flashed on and off within the receptive field.

6. Some directions of stimulus movement across the receptive field are far more effective in evoking impulses than are others.

7. Slowly moving targets generally evoke more impulses than do rapidly moving stimuli.

8. Repeated presention of the same stimulus produces response habituation.

This complex of receptive field properties is particularly well suited to underlie attentive and orientation behaviors. The neurons are most responsive to the kinds of novel, moving stimuli that preferentially elicit attention and orientation (or defense), and they code the parameters of

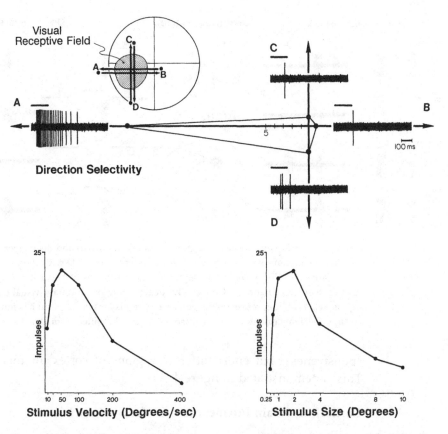

Figure 4.4 A visually responsive deep-layer neuron. The schematic in the upper left indicates the position of the neuron's receptive field and the paths of stimulus movement. Nasal-to-temporal movement (B-to-A) was strongly preferred, as shown in the polar coordinate plot of average number of impulses evoked by the different directions of movement (each cross hatch = one impulse). As shown by the graphs at the bottom, this neuron responded best to small (2°) stimuli moved at low (50°/sec) velocities.

movement (e.g., direction and velocity) that are necessary for predicting the location of a moving target to intercept or avoid it (figure 4.4).

In order for superior colliculus neurons to achieve their characteristic complement of receptive field features, a higher-order visual cortex influence is critical. Moreover, this corticotectal influence is likely to be necessary to ensure that superior colliculus activity can be modified and modulated by experience and current needs. In this way the effectiveness of a given stimulus in evoking superior colliculus-mediated behaviors can change, depending on the state of the organism and the context within which the stimulus appears. This corticotectal influence is impressively powerful, and temporarily deactivating it by reversible cooling can eliminate even vigorous responses in many superior colliculus neurons. It is interesting to note that both superficial- and deep-layer visual neurons depend on corticotectal influences for much of their re-

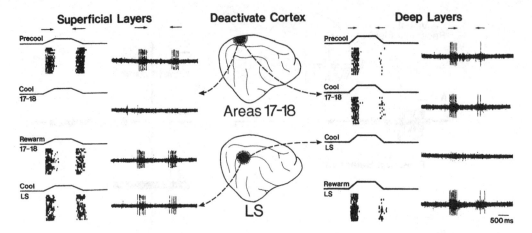

Figure 4.5 Cortex controls visual responses. Both superficial- and deep-layer neurons are strongly dependent on visual cortex, but on different areas. Deactivating primary visual cortex (areas 17–18) by cooling it depresses the responses of superficial layer neurons, but not deep-layer neurons. Conversely, deactivating extraprimary visual cortex (lateral suprasylvian, LS) depresses the responses of deep layer neurons and has minimal effects on superficial-layer neurons (in this case no effect). (Modified from Ogasawara et al. 1984)

sponsiveness, but enlist different regions of cortex for this purpose. This is demonstrated in figure 4.5.

Cortical-Midbrain Interactions and the Sprague Effect

Today there is much less emphasis on relating overt behavior to differences between the receptive field properties of cortical and superior colliculus neurons, and a growing emphasis on the extensive interactions among them to produce normal vision in both mammalian and nonmammalian species (Sprague 1966a,b; Schneider 1969; Ingle 1973b; Webster 1974; Jassik-Gerschenfeld and Hardy 1984; Ewert 1984; Hardy and Stein 1988). Perhaps the most dramatic example of the delicate balance among related components of the visual system was provided by Sprague in 1966. In a deceptively simple and very clever experiment, Sprague used the cat's natural propensity to orient to novel stimuli to map its normal visual field, or "food perimetry" (Kluver 1937). He then used that map to assess the effect on visually guided behavior of large posterior neocortical lesions that destroyed all of visual cortex and its surrounding tissue as well. A normal cat will orient to stimuli anywhere within 90 to 105 degrees of fixation. However, after experiencing a large lesion of, for example, the right cortex, a previously normal cat showed a profound visual neglect of the left, or contralateral visual field (figure 4.6). This neglect looked very much like that seen after a lesion of the superior colliculus, even though the superior colliculus itself remained intact. However, following removal of the superior colliculus on the side opposite the cortical lesion (in this case the left superior colliculus),

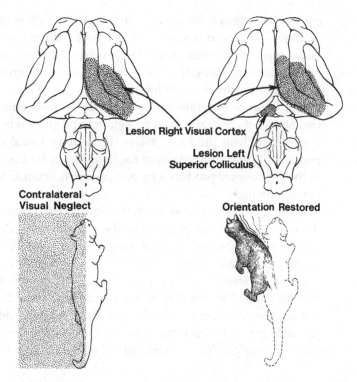

Lesion Right Visual Cortex

Lesion Left
Superior Colliculus

Contralateral
Visual Neglect

Orientation Restored

Figure 4.6 The Sprague effect. Behavioral deficits induced by ipsilateral cortical lesions can be reversed by lesioning the contralateral superior colliculus. Destruction of visual cortices on the right produces inattention to cues in the left visual field. Ablation of the left superior colliculus restores these orienting responses.

the defect was reversed. Now the animal's orienting behavior to stimuli in the previously impaired left hemifield appeared to be normal—a dramatic demonstration of the amelioration of a lesion-induced deficit by a second lesion.

The explanation for the Sprague effect lies in the fact that the superior colliculus depends a great deal on inputs from visual cortex for its processing of visual information. In the absence of cortical input, superior colliculus neurons are usually more difficult to excite and lack many of their complex features (e.g., direction selectivity, binocularity). Excitatory cortical inputs are derived from the ipsilateral cortex (Ogasawara et al. 1984) and are counterbalanced by contralateral inhibitory inputs (Hoffmann and Straschill 1971; Goodale 1973; Saraiva et al. 1978) derived from substantia nigra and transmitted through the commissure connecting the left and right superior colliculi (Wallace et al. 1989, 1990). When visual cortex (e.g., right) was lesioned in these experiments, the right superior colliculus became dominated by inhibitory inputs from substantia nigra traveling through the intercollicular commissure. Eliminating commissural-mediated inhibitory inputs by either lesioning the left superior colliculus (Sprague 1966a; Hardy and Stein 1988) or cutting the commissure (Sherman 1974a) restored a balance to the system and allowed the right superior colliculus to regain some of its function. Its neurons still lacked many of the properties normally derived from the visual cortex and undoubtedly lost much of their information processing capabilities; nevertheless, they functioned well enough to underlie gross attentive and orientation responses. These observations point out the importance of symmetry between the two superior colliculi and the two halves of the brain, thereby helping to explain why removal of both superior colliculi produces a less devastating visual dysfunction than removal of one: compensation for their loss is far easier in the absence of the asymmetry produced by pairing one functional and one nonfunctional structure.

It is not necessary to remove the entire visual cortex to compromise the integrity of visual neurons in the superior colliculus and produce a neglect of contralateral visual space. All cortical visual areas do not contribute equally to the properties of the deep-layer visual neurons involved in attentive and orientation behaviors, and a particularly important cortical area has now been identified in the posterior aspect of the suprasylvian cortex (Hardy and Stein 1988). Lesions as small as a few millimeters in this extrastriate area alter the properties of deep layer neurons and produce a contralateral visual neglect (figure 4.7) that is

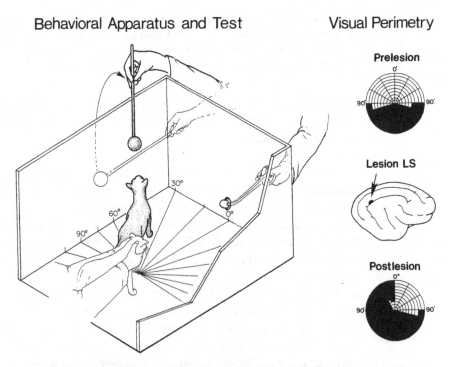

Figure 4.7 Very small lesions in LS induce visual neglect. A normal cat will orient to a visual stimulus anywhere from fixation (0°) to more than 90° to either side. This is its visual field, or perimetry (prelesion). A small lesion (black spot) in the posterior portion of LS disrupts corticotectal influences on the ipsilateral superior colliculus and produces a complete contralateral visual neglect (postlesion). (Modified from Hardy and Stein 1988)

also readily reversed by removing the inputs passing through the opposite superior colliculus. The dependence of deep-layer neurons on extra-primary cortical inputs for their normal response properties will be shown to be typical of each of the sensory modalities represented here. Presumably, these anatomical and physiological similarities across modalities reflect common mechanisms for subserving similar overt responses to different stimuli.

Auditory, Somatosensory, and Nociceptive Involvement of the Superior Colliculus

Because of the tremendous volume of information that had been gathered about the superior colliculus—the eye movements produced by its activation, the visual anomalies produced by its destruction, and the visual properties of its constituent neurons—the view of the superior colliculus as an exclusively visual structure persisted for some time (and continues to pop up in some quarters today). Even the appearance of some early anatomical reports describing substantial nonvisual afferents to its deeper aspects (Walker 1942, 1943; Marburg and Warner 1947; Poirier and Bertrand 1955; Anderson and Berry 1959; Mehler et al. 1960) and early suggestions that it might play a role in somesthesis and even pain did little to dispel this notion.

It is curious to note that as late as 1962 the deeper layers were described as containing "cells that respond to extraoptic stimulation of unknown origin" (Altman and Malis 1962). However, within a few years, reports began to appear showing that these deeper layers contain neurons responsive to somatosensory and auditory stimuli as well as to visual stimuli (Bell et al. 1964; Jassik-Gerschenfeld 1965; Horn and Hill 1966). These neurons are not simply providing crude signals that somatosensory or auditory stimuli are present; over time it has become apparent that the nonvisual response properties of superior colliculus neurons have selectivities for stimulus features that rival those of neighboring visually responsive neurons.

AUDITORY INVOLVEMENT

Receptive Field Properties of Auditory Neurons

The contrasting properties and organizations of auditory neurons in the superior colliculus and along the auditory thalamocortical system are readily apparent even with casual observation. Neurons in the primary auditory pathways are particularly well suited to discriminate pure tones (i.e., sounds composed of a single frequency), and neurons with similar tonal sensitivities, or "isofrequencies," are arranged in bands in primary auditory cortex to produce a "tonotopic" map (Reale and Imig 1980), but no map of auditory space has been found here. In contrast, auditory neurons in the superior colliculus are comparatively insensitive to pure tones, being more specialized for signaling the spatial location of sounds than for identifying their spectral compositions. They prefer complex sounds composed of multiple frequencies, like those produced by jangling keys, hisses, hand claps (Horn and Hill 1966; Wickelgren 1971; Stein and Arigbede 1972; Gordon 1973; Graham et al. 1981), and by the vocalizations of conspecifics (Mast and Chung 1973). They respond best to moving stimuli, and some even exhibit directional selectivity (Gordon 1973; Rauschecker and Harris 1989). Unlike auditory neurons elsewhere in the nervous system, they habituate if stimuli are presented repeatedly, and are therefore best suited for detecting novel sounds. They also have broad tuning curves that are biased toward the higher frequencies and have higher-than-average thresholds (Mast and Chung 1973; Wise and Irvine 1983; Hirsch et al. 1985).

Most significant is the ability of these neurons, nearly all of which are binaural, to compare differences in the physical properties of the stimuli picked up by the two ears. They are exquisitely sensitive to differences in the temporal interval (interaural time difference) and intensity (interaural intensity difference) of these inputs. Sounds to the left of the midline are louder and arrive earlier at the left ear because they are not shadowed by the head, effects which are exaggerated in elephants and minimized in mice as a result of the vast differences in the sizes of their heads.

By systematically varying interaural intensity differences via separate speakers placed in each ear, Wise and Irvine (1983, 1985) and Hirsch and associates (1985) showed that there are several binaural categories of auditory neurons in cat superior colliculus. Wise and Irvine identified each by a three letter code. Of four neuronal types, the most common EO/I, is excited by inputs from the contralateral ear (E), does not respond to inputs from the ipsilateral ear alone (O), and exhibits antagonism or inhibition between the two ears (I) when they are stimulated together (obviously, the ipsilateral input is inhibitory). In contrast, in the other three categories, facilitation (F) occurs among inputs from the two ears: EE/F neurons respond to either ear alone, but better to their combination; EO/F neurons respond to the contralateral ear alone, do not respond to the ipsilateral ear alone, and are facilitated by stimulation of the two ears together; OO/F neurons respond to neither ear alone, but do respond to their combined inputs.

By integrating inputs from the two ears, most auditory neurons in the superior colliculus construct spatially restricted receptive fields (King and Palmer 1983, 1985; Middlebrooks and Knudsen 1984; Middlebrooks 1987) with internal nonhomogeneities in excitability and clearly defined regions of maximal response called "best areas." The

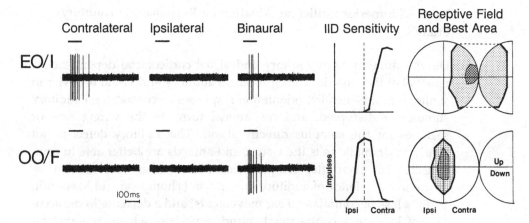

Contralateral   Ipsilateral   Binaural   IID Sensitivity   Receptive Field and Best Area

EO/I

OO/F

100ms

Impulses

Ipsi   Contra   Ipsi   Contra

Up
Down

Figure 5.1 Auditory receptive fields are based on inputs from both ears. EO/I type neurons show excitatory responses to a contralateral stimulus (E), no response to an ipsilateral stimulus (O), and inhibition (I) when both stimuli (binaural) are presented. These neurons prefer interaural intensity differences (IID sensitivities) that favor the contralateral side and, correspondingly, have contralateral receptive fields. This EO/I receptive field extended beyond 90° contralateral and is illustrated on a diagram in which the auditory area from 90–180° contralateral is folded forward in order to make it visible here. In contrast, OO/F type neurons show no responses to either ear alone (monaural cues), and respond only when the interaural intensity differences between the two ears are negligible. Such a neuron has its receptive field in frontal auditory space. The "best area" (inner stippled area) within an auditory receptive field is that region from which >75% of the maximum response is evoked.

exception is the EE/F type, which will respond to stimuli anywhere in auditory space. EO/F and OO/F types have receptive fields whose centers, or best areas, are within 20 degrees of the frontal midline (figure 5.1), and EO/I neurons have receptive fields restricted to portions of the contralateral hemifield. Because the EO/I type is restricted by inhibition from the ipsilateral ear, its contralateral excitatory region is flanked by a largely ipsilateral inhibitory zone (figure 5.1).

Corticotectal Influences on Auditory Neurons

The source of corticotectal auditory inputs is the area in the anterior ectosylvian sulcus known as Field AES (FAES in figure 3.2), a region which has neither a tonotopic nor a spatiotopic organization (Clarey and Irvine 1986, 1990). Removal of this corticotectal input depresses the auditory activity of superior colliculus neurons and raises their thresholds so that louder sounds are necessary to drive them (Meredith and Clemo 1989); however, their basic interaural and receptive field characteristics remain unaltered. This contrasts with the visual system and reflects different dependencies among sensory representations in the superior colliculus on ascending and descending inputs.

Effect of Superior Colliculus Ablation on Responses to Auditory Stimuli

Despite differences in auditory and visual corticotectal dependencies, removal of the superior colliculus alters auditory and visual behavior in similar ways. Generally, orientation responses to contralateral auditory stimuli are disrupted, and the animal turns to the wrong side or searches for the stimulus directly ahead. The auditory defect is not nearly as dramatic as is the visual, and animals are better able to compensate. But even after compensation there remains a persistent increase in the latency of auditory orientation (Thompson and Masterton 1978), a loss of contralateral ear movements, and a decrease in the accuracy of locating a contralateral sound, especially when presented far from the midline (Sprague and Meikle 1965). Bilateral lesions are far less disruptive on auditory behaviors than unilateral lesions (as on visual behaviors, see above); persistent defects in response to auditory (or visual) stimuli are minimal and reflect the animal's lack of head movements to stimuli in upper space. Thus, auditory compensation is easiest to accomplish when midbrain lesions are symmetrical. It would be interesting to see if contralateral auditory deficits would be caused by unilateral ablation of Field AES, and if they could be ameliorated by sectioning the intercollicular commissure. If so, it would demonstrate a fundamental similarity with the organization of superior colliculus-mediated auditory and visual behaviors, a parallel that is generally assumed to be present.

SOMATOSENSORY INVOLVEMENT

Receptive Field Properties of Somatosensory Neurons

As described in the discussion of afferent pathways, somatosensory information can reach the superior colliculus by a variety of routes, and there are many neurons in the superior colliculus responsive to stimulation of the body. Although some of these somatosensory-responsive neurons require the distortion of subcutaneous tissue, most respond well to stimulation of the hair and/or skin and have well-defined receptive fields (Stein and Arigbede 1972). The response properties of these neurons have been compared to the mechanoreceptor types described in peripheral somatosensory afferents and appear to preserve many of their characteristics (Stein et al. 1976b; Nagata and Kruger 1979). Many respond well to low-velocity stimuli, but most prefer intermediate- or high-velocity stimuli and will fail to respond even to forceful stimuli if they are presented very gradually.

Regardless of the velocity requirements of the different neuronal types, all respond in transient, or rapidly adapting fashion, even to maintained stimuli. They most closely resemble the intermediate- and

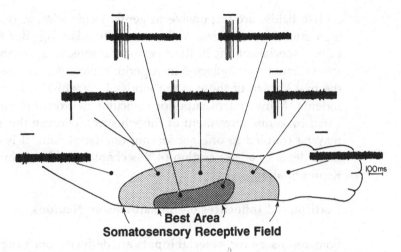

Best Area
Somatosensory Receptive Field

Figure 5.2 Internal organization of a somatosensory receptive field. This receptive field was located on the distal forelimb. Some points within the receptive field were more effective than others, and the "best area" (>75% of maximum response) was near the center.

high-velocity hair (G intermediate and G1) and skin (F intermediate and F1) receptor categories described by Burgess (1973) for first-order afferents. However, unlike peripheral afferents, but very much like the deep layer visual and auditory neurons, they habituate rather rapidly to somatosensory stimuli presented at high iterative rates. Thus, they seem best suited to dealing with the novel stimuli that usually elicit attentive and orientation responses (Stein et al. 1976b; Clemo and Stein 1984, 1986; Nagata and Kruger 1979).

Somatosensory receptive fields follow the same pattern as their neighboring visual and auditory receptive fields: they are large and, like auditory receptive fields, are nonhomogeneous, with clearly defined best regions (Clemo and Stein 1991). An example is illustrated in figure 5.2. Progressively larger stimuli within the best region evoke progressively higher numbers of impulses. Surprisingly, however, comparatively few of these neurons exhibit the suppressive surrounds or directional selectivity (Clemo and Stein 1987) characteristic of the visual and auditory representations. Although direction selectivity and surround inhibition are present in somatosensory cortical neurons, they are far less common in the somatosensory system than in the visual system. Whether differences in modality-specific properties of superior colliculus neurons reflect different modes of resolving spatial characteristics and direction of movement in these modalities or simply the absence of such coding in the somatosensory representation in superior colliculus neurons remains to be determined.

The fundamental receptive field characteristics of somatosensory neurons described here for the cat superior colliculus are generally reflective of those in other species as well: most have comparatively large receptive fields, are responsive to gentle tactile stimuli, respond best to high stimulus velocities, and are rapidly adapting. But many species exhibit specializations in their peripheral sensory apparatus, and these specializations are reflected in superior colliculus organization. Perhaps the best known of these is the vibrissal, or whisker, representation in rodents. Many rodent superior colliculus neurons are vigorously activated by gentle movement of the whiskers. Because this specialization may be coupled to one subserving oral-facial pain, it is dealt with in more detail in a later section of this chapter entitled Pain (Nociceptive) Representation.

Corticotectal Influences on Somatosensory Neurons

Somatosensory corticotectal inputs are derived from a region in the anterior ectosylvian cortex called SIV. The inputs from SIV, like the cortical inputs to visual and auditory neurons, are almost exclusively excitatory. Removing them depresses the responses of superior colliculus neurons to tactile stimuli (Clemo and Stein 1986). The dependence of somatosensory neurons on cortex lies somewhere in between that exhibited by visual and auditory neurons. That is, cortical (SIV) removal does more than simply raise the activation thresholds of somatosensory neurons, as is the case in the auditory representation; however, unlike visual neurons, no specific receptive field characteristic depends on somatosensory cortical input. Furthermore, far more somatosensory neurons are unaffected by corticotectal deactivation than are their visual counterparts. It is obvious that while the different sensory representations in the superior colliculus show striking parallels in overall organization, they are not simply copies of one another.

Effects of Superior Colliculus Ablation on Responses to Somatosensory Stimuli

Immediately after unilateral superior colliculus lesions, animals lose their ability to respond appropriately to touch on the contralateral body (Sprague and Meikle 1965; also see Casagrande et al. 1972), particularly on the caudal body regions. The deficits are manifested as either an absence of a reaction, or a reaction directed to the wrong part of the body. In some instances touching the contralateral foot will produce a turning to the ipsilateral side. The animals compensate for these attentive and orientation deficits over the course of the first postsurgical month, until the only gross defects remaining are in response to stimulation of the contralateral hindlimb. While it is tantalizing to speculate about how this compensation comes about (and it does seem like a critical question), too little is known about the mechanisms by which these tasks are relearned and the areas of the brain that accomplish it.

As in the case of vision and audition, bilaterally symmetrical lesions are far less disruptive to somatosensory behavior than are unilateral lesions and, with the exception of difficulty in dealing with stimuli on its back or the top of its head, no persistent gross defects have been noted.

The same questions based on the visual system that were raised in the section on auditory representation are germane here: Would depriving the superior colliculus of its somatosensory corticotectal input produce somatosensory deficits similar to those incurred by superior colliculus lesions? If so, would these deficits be ameliorated by removing inputs from the opposite superior colliculus? In short, just how closely do the functional organizations of the different sensory modalities parallel one another?

PAIN (NOCICEPTIVE) REPRESENTATION

An early indication that the superior colliculus might be involved in pain comes from a report published in 1943 by Walker. He believed that pain was integrated at three levels: cortex, thalamus, and tectum mesencephali (the roof of the midbrain and composed of the superior and inferior colliculi). Walker came to this conclusion after noting that lesions of the spinothalamic tract at the level of the midbrain (the region of the brachium of the inferior colliculus) produced temporary analgesia in patients, presumably by depriving the midbrain of fibers carrying information about noxious stimuli. While many of these spinothalamic fibers were certainly en route to a variety of midbrain regions, including the superior colliculus, and while the spinothalamic pathway undoubtedly contains fibers capable of carrying information about noxious stimuli, there was no way to know if the postsurgical analgesia was due specifically to disruption of nociceptive fibers destined to terminate in either of the colliculi. It may have been due to disruption of fibers that were simply passing through this region on their way to more rostral pain-processing areas. Furthermore, Walker himself emphasized the inferior, rather than the superior, colliculus.

Other early observations in man and animal subjects could also be interpreted as pointing to a role for the superior colliculus in pain, although these, too, had problems of interpretation due to the possibility of involving fibers destined for other structures (Reyes et al. 1951; Spiegal et al. 1954; Nashold et al. 1969; Delgado 1965). There are semantic problems inherent in defining what is painful in different individuals, and there are problems in quantitatively defining stimuli that will be painful in all circumstances to all subjects. To avoid these problems, the terms *nociceptive* and *nociception*, which lack the psychological connotations of the term *pain*, are usually preferred (Zimmermann 1976) and will be used below.

Receptive Field Properties of Nociceptive Neurons

It was not until 1978 that the first direct evidence was presented for the involvement of superior colliculus neurons in nociception (Stein and Dixon 1978). In this study superior colliculus neurons were observed to respond to noxious mechanical and/or thermal stimuli. Some of these neurons clearly were multisensory and were responsive to visual, innocuous tactile, and noxious somatic stimuli. Their responses to noxious stimuli appeared to be very much like those of nociceptive neurons of the dorsal horn of the spinal cord: one group required frankly noxious stimuli to evoke responses (nociceptive-specific, NS), and the other was activated by low-threshold mechanical stimuli but responded with more impulses and at a higher frequency by either noxious mechanical or noxious thermal stimuli (wide dynamic range, WDR) (figure 5.3). Thus, the same two types of nociceptive neurons found in the dorsal horn were represented in the superior colliculus. The nociceptive responses of both NS and WDR superior colliculus neurons were blocked by opiates, and this opiate block was readily reversed by the opiate antagonist naloxone, just as in the spinal cord and thalamus. A detailed, quantitative follow-up study of these neurons in the hamster showed that their receptive fields and stimulus-response profiles are very similar to those of the NS and WDR neurons studied in the spinal cord, thalamus, and higher brain centers of other species (Larson et al. 1987). Even the exponents of the stimulus-response functions for individual and groups of neurons are strikingly similar to those described in various areas of the central nervous system of other rodents and even primates. Like cutaneous and auditory receptive fields, many nociceptive neurons (i.e., WDR) have central best zones, surrounded by areas of lowered sensitivity.

The presence of the same two classes of nociceptive neurons in the superior colliculus (WDR and NS) and in other structures involved in nociception as well as the striking similarities in their properties are not a result of all structures sharing the same sets of afferents. Some projections from laminae I (where NS neurons abound) and V (where many WDR neurons are found) of the medullary dorsal horn are shared by thalamus and superior colliculus, but shared inputs constitute only a minority of the projections to these structures (Bruce et al. 1987). Furthermore, the patterns of descending afferent inputs among central nervous system structures with nociceptive neurons are quite diverse. Thus, their similar response properties do not reflect a duplication of input systems, but rather a fundamental constancy of both WDR and NS neurons at all levels of the central nervous system that occurs despite very different afferent pathways (McHaffie et al. 1989; Price et al. 1992). Although there are some differences in the sizes of nociceptive receptive fields in different structures, the information processing capabilities of NS and WDR neurons in the dorsal horn of the spinal cord,

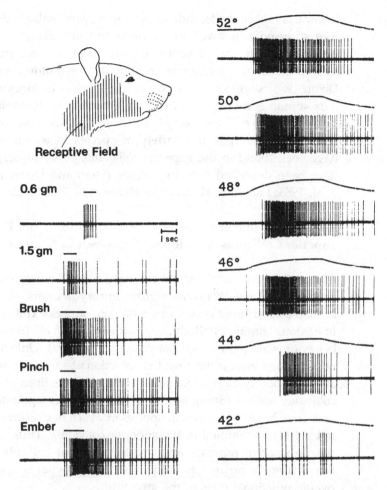

Figure 5.3 A wide-dynamic range neuron from a rat superior colliculus. A restricted area of the cheek and neck was sensitive to innocuous (a 0.6-gm brush or a 1.5-gm brush that indented the skin) as well as to noxious (pinch, ember) stimuli. Responses were graded according to stimulus intensity. Vigorous and long-lasting responses were evoked by noxious thermal stimuli (52–46°C), but weak and phasic responses were evoked by innocuous thermal stimuli (44–42°C). The ramp-like trace above each oscillogram indicates the increasing and decreasing temperature of the thermal stimulus. The maximum temperature reached is indicated. (From McHaffie et al. 1989)

medullary dorsal horn, and thalamus are indistinguishable from those of NS and WDR neurons in the superior colliculus. It appears as if comparatively little transformation of information takes place as nociceptive signals are moved from one place to another in the brain. This lends credence to a notion that structures containing WDR and NS neurons do what they do as a consequence of the targets to which they project, not as a consequence of dealing differently with incoming signals. This situation is quite similar to that for visual neurons in superficial versus deep layers of the superior colliculus discussed earlier.

The presence of nociceptive neurons in the superior colliculus of mammals makes sense; indeed, it would seem maladaptive for a structure so heavily involved in attentive and orientation behaviors to be unresponsive to the presence of potentially harmful stimuli. That at least some of these neurons in rodents are multisensory (Stein and Dixon 1978) suggests that information about both innocuous and noxious stimuli is integrated in the same circuits to determine the appropriate response. This would seem to be adaptive in all species; nevertheless, despite the variety of species in which nonvisual cells have been found in the superior colliculus, so far nociceptive neurons have been described only in rodents (Stein and Dixon 1978; Rhoades et al. 1983; Larson et al. 1987; McHaffie et al. 1989; Aury et al. 1991).

Corticotectal Influences on Nociceptive Neurons, and Effects of Superior Colliculus Ablation on Responses to Noxious Stimuli

Although corticotectal influences have been demonstrated on visual, auditory, and low-threshold somatosensory neurons, no information is available about how cortex can modulate superior colliculus responses to noxious stimuli. Similarly, very little is known about how nociceptive behavior is altered by superior colliculus removal. Only a few scattered observations exist indicating that reactions to noxious stimuli become atypical, poorly organized, and sometimes misdirected after superior colliculus lesions (Sprague and Meikle 1965; Casagrande et al. 1972), and these have been made in species in which nociceptive neurons have not yet been identified in the superior colliculus. Thus, the purpose of the nociceptive representation in the superior colliculus must be inferred from its organizational properties and what is known about the overall functional roles of the structure.

Role of the Nociceptive Representation in the Superior Colliculus

The nociceptive representation in the rodent superior colliculus is a selective one that is biased to responding to stimulation of the face (McHaffie et al. 1989). While many of the nociceptive neurons have receptive fields that include the forelimb, comparatively few have been found that respond to stimulation of more caudal body parts. This seems particularly appropriate in animals that make extensive use of their whiskers for exploration, for unlike the eyes or ears, the whiskers operate only at short distances so the face and forelimbs are put at maximal risk during the animal's normal exploratory behavior. Presumably, activation of superior colliculus nociceptive neurons will serve an immediate protective function by initiating withdrawal responses (figure 5.4) in most circumstances. There is now substantial evidence from studies using chemical and electrical stimulation of the superior colliculus in rodents (Redgrave et al. 1981; Sahibzada et al. 1986; Ellard and Goodale 1986, 1988; Dean et al. 1988a,b) that withdrawal as well as

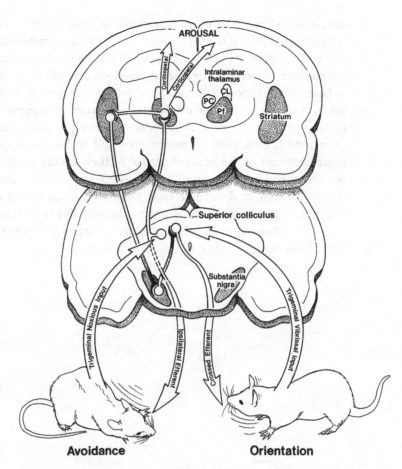

Avoidance   **Orientation**

Figure 5.4 The presumptive circuit underlying superior colliculus–mediated approach/ avoidance. Shown here is the initiation of orientation behaviors via the activation of whisker-responsive neurons, and avoidance behavior via the activation of nociceptive-responsive neurons. These two neuronal populations exert their influences through different pathways: orientation by the crossed tecto-reticulo-spinal pathway, and avoidance via the ipsilateral descending bundle. Innocuous and noxious inputs from the face may also interact in output neurons to ensure that when the face contacts potentially damaging stimuli, orientation responses are actively suppressed (via a pathway involving the parafascicularis [Pf] nucleus, the striatum, and the substantia nigra). Inhibitory synapses are shown in black. (PC, paracentral nucleus; CL, central lateral nucleus. Modified from McHaffie et al. 1989)

approach responses can be evoked, and that these opposing tendencies are mediated by two different descending pathways (the ipsilateral efferent bundle for withdrawal and the medial crossed efferent, or predorsal, bundle for approach; see figures 3.3 and 5.4). The observation that the sites from which electrically evoked withdrawal responses are initiated are the same sites at which nociceptive neurons are located prompted McHaffie and co-workers (1989) to postulate that noxious stimuli activate nociceptive superior colliculus neurons to produce withdrawal. Presumably, at least some nociceptive superior colliculus neurons will be shown to project primarily or exclusively in the ipsilateral efferent bundle by which withdrawal behaviors are mediated. However, other nociceptive neurons may project via the predorsal bundle to initiate an orientation to a persistently noxious stimulus.

These observations are consistent with a role for the superior colliculus in nociception, and presumably a nociceptive representation is not unique to the rodent. If it is present in the primate, one would also expect its organization to be maplike and to have a disproportionate representation of the hands because of their involvement in tactile exploration and manipulation. Yet, regardless of species considerations, it is of interest to determine how noxious stimuli, which are normally prepotent, modulate (and/or are modulated by) the other sensory inputs to multisensory superior colliculus neurons and how these physiological interactions relate to overt behaviors.

III   Multiple, Overlapping Sensory and Motor Maps

REPRESENTING SENSORY SPACE

A problem shared by all nervous systems is how to represent a given expanse of peripheral sensory tissue. The problem is multifaceted, and at least two requirements in the solution, which seem to be present across a range of sensory modalities, deserve mention here. First, the representation must be easy to produce and modify during early development. This allows it to conform to growth-induced changes in the body and in the peripheral sensory organ, and allows it to conform to experience-induced changes in the use of that sensory organ; a requirement that extends to motor systems as well. (Developmental issues that relate to multisensory integration will be dealt with in part IV.) Second, it must follow systematic organizational rules sufficiently rigorous that the essential features of the peripheral stimulus, such as what it is and where it is in space, will be identified unequivocally by patterns and sites of central activity. It is this second issue, especially the part about identifying where the stimulus is, that turns out to be most germane to what has been learned about the spatial factors involved in multisensory integration.

A common solution to the problem of how to represent sensory space is the construction of a maplike re-creation of the receptor epithelium and, thus, of the sensory space it serves. However, as will be described below, the auditory map is based on a computation of the inputs arriving at the two ears rather than the more direct spatial reconstruction of the receptor surface like that evident in the visual and somatosensory systems. Nevertheless, the issue here remains the same for each of these representations.

At each successive level in the central nervous system the visual, somatosensory, and auditory representations occupy spatially distinct regions that are defined functionally and anatomically (i.e., cytoarchitectonically). At the cortical level, and in most regions of the thalamus, the domain of an individual sensory modality consists of distinct maps. The map (or maps) of a single sensory modality in, for example, primary sensory cortex is distinguished from the map in extraprimary cortex it abuts by mirror-image reversals in receptive field progressions, significant changes in receptive field properties, differences in afferent/efferent organization, and/or by specialization for different submodality characteristics. In cortex the interposition of "association" areas further segregates the representations of the different sensory modalities.

The discovery that sensory and motor representations are distributed in maplike form has been of tremendous value in understanding general principles of brain organization. It has also been an extremely useful tool for studying how the brain develops during prenatal and early postnatal life. But once one begins to deal with more complex sensorimotor issues than those related to the production of reflexes, the outer limits of our understanding of the manner in which this principle is translated into function are quickly reached. How the brain recognizes which areas of its sensory maps are activated so that it can infer stimulus location in the outside world and how it recognizes which areas of its motor maps need to be activated to produce a particular movement to respond to that stimulus are enduring mysteries. At present, it is not even clear how to formulate the experimental questions that would help us come to grips with such issues.

Nevertheless, it is reasonable to suppose that segregating the different sensory maps from one another is a simple way to avoid confusion among modalities, and using submodality features to separate maps within each modality is one way to facilitate the coding and recognition of certain stimulus characteristics. For example, the effect of a stimulus is localized not only to the appropriate maps, but to a specific area within each map. The individual map most activated depends on how closely the response properties of its constituent neurons match the physical characteristics of a particular stimulus.

THE SUPERIOR COLLICULUS

That the superior colliculus does not follow the eminently reasonable pattern found elsewhere in the central nervous system seems surprising at first. Its unimodal visual, auditory, and somatosensory neurons are intermixed with multisensory neurons in its deep layers, with no uninterrupted sheet of tissue devoted to any single sensory representation or to any submodality feature. A description of the sensory maps in the superior colliculus is provided in chapter 6.

The reason for this deviation from the common organizational plan, so orderly in the primary projection nuclei, is probably a direct reflection of the involvement of all of these sensory systems and submodality features in the behavioral roles of the structure; that is, the superior colliculus does not separate among its inputs in the standard way because its job is one of integrating, not segregating, the modalities.

SENSORIMOTOR TRANSFORMATION AND MOTOR ORGANIZATION

The attentive and orientation roles of the superior colliculus involve the pooling of sensory inputs to redirect the very organs from which these inputs originate (e.g., eyes, ears, head) in order to localize, or capture (and in some cases to avoid), the source of the stimulus. It is by virtue of the convergence and intermixing of sensory inputs that efficiency is achieved in giving different sensory modalities access to the same motor output circuits (Stein et al. 1976b). In this way, any and all of the sensory modalities represented can direct any and all of the peripheral sensory organs from which sensory inputs are derived. Each of the motor organizations in the deep superior colliculus can be viewed independently in the same way that the sensory maps can be viewed independently. Yet, in building this convenient scheme for sensorimotor transduction the nervous system appears to have used a simple alignment of the different sensory and motor maps, often making multiple use of the same neurons (i.e., many of the same neurons respond to multiple sensory inputs and some are premotor efferents as well). These relationships are, then, interdependent. These issues are dealt with in the chapters in this part as well as those in part IV. First, each of the sensory and motor maps is examined individually, as are the evolutionary constancies in them that are believed to be reflected by organizational parallels among mammalian and nonmammalian species. Then, in part IV the interactions among sensory modalities are stressed, and it is suggested that the various sensory and motor maps can be viewed as components of a larger integrated entity.

6　Sensory Maps

SUPERFICIAL-LAYER VISUAL REPRESENTATION

It has been known for some time that the visual organization in the superficial layers of the superior colliculus in cat, and all other species examined, is maplike or *visuotopic* (e.g., cat: Apter 1945; Feldon et al. 1970; Berman and Cynader 1972; rabbit: Schaefer 1970; monkey: Cynader and Berman 1972; guinea pig: King and Palmer 1983; hamster: Finlay et al. 1978; rat: Siminoff et al. 1966; mouse: Drager and Hubel 1976; opossum: Volchan et al. 1978). Although deep-layer visual neurons exist, until recently whenever the visual map of the superior colliculus has been discussed in the literature, it has been this superficial-layer representation to which reference has been made. As in other visual structures, the map is constructed by plotting the positions of receptive fields (primarily their centers) found along a vertical electrode penetration and then comparing the clusters of receptive fields found along penetrations made in different locations in the structure. The resultant visuotopy in every species is elegant in its simplicity: neurons whose receptive fields are nasal in visual space are located rostral, and those with temporal visual fields are represented caudally (e.g., Kruger 1970; Stein 1981). Therefore, the representation of the horizontal meridian of visual space runs from the front of the structure to the rear. Similarly, the representation of the vertical meridian of visual space is oriented along the medial to lateral aspect (figure 6.1).

This representation is a fundamental vertebrate plan, but one in which substantial species variations exist in terms of the presence and magnitude of a geometric expansion of the central visual field, and the representation of one or two eyes in the same superior colliculus (for further discussion, see Stein and Meredith 1990). Many species do not exhibit a simple linear transformation of the retina or visual field in the maps constructed in their superior colliculi. Rather, the maps directly reflect the animals' visual behaviors. Cats, monkeys, and many other animals, including man, make heavy use of their central retinas in fixating and examining objects of interest, and there is a corresponding

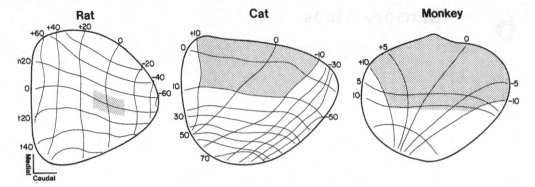

Figure 6.1 Visual maps in superficial layers. The horizontal meridians (nasal-temporal in visual space) run rostral-caudal and the vertical meridians (superior-inferior) run medial-lateral (minus signs refer to positions in inferior visual space). The stippling denotes the representation of the central 10° of the visual field. Note the differing geometric expansions of central vision (shading) in the different species. Also note that the 0° vertical meridian (which marks the division of the visual field into ipsilateral and contralateral components) in the rat is near the center of the structure, so that the rostral half represents much of the ipsilateral or nasal (n) visual field and the caudal half represents contralateral or temporal (t) visual space. In the cat only the representation in the rostral pole of the structure extends (10°) into the ipsilateral field, and the representation in the monkey ends at the vertical meridian. (The maps are taken from studies by Siminoff et al. 1966 [rat], Feldon et al. 1970, with permission from Pergamon Press Ltd. [cat] and Cynader and Berman 1972 [rhesus monkey].)

increase in the amount of tissue devoted to representing this region of the retina (figure 6.1).

DEEP-LAYER VISUAL REPRESENTATION

The receptive fields of deep layer visual neurons are far larger than those of superficial-layer neurons. This difference becomes apparent as soon as an electrode descending through the superior colliculus reaches below the stratum opticum, the lower border of the superficial layers. Now, in the deep aspects of the superior colliculus, visual receptive fields exhibit an abrupt change in size, and average a fourfold increment in diameter from those of the superficial layers. Furthermore, as the electrode advances through the tissue, receptive field centers vary considerably with respect to one another, sometimes shifting erratically within the same vertical column of tissue (Meredith and Stein 1990). This is rarely found in the superficial layers. These observations indicate that the deep-layer visual representation is not a simple extension of the superficial map. In fact, superficial–deep layer differences in receptive field size and the spatial fidelity of receptive field centers within the same electrode penetration make the mapping techniques used in detailing the superficial-layer visuotopy seem inappropriate in deep layers. A standard map, dependent on the positions of receptive field centers, like that used superficially (as well as in the geniculocortical system), would fail to deal with the fact that while the centers of large deep-layer receptive fields are often out of register with each other, much of the area of their receptive fields is overlapping. A map of receptive field centers would also seriously underestimate the extent of the superior colliculus activated by a single point in visual space.

To detail the deep-layer map, it was most advantageous to use a method that determines the areas of visual space that have access to the same region (i.e., a "point-image"; see McIlwain 1975). Put another way, this technique determines how much of the superior colliculus is activated by a single point somewhere in visual space, and therefore examines how much of the structure "sees" the same point. Determining the map in this way made it obvious that comparatively large blocks of tissue represent the same points in visual space (Meredith and Stein 1990). As one would expect in a map, the block of tissue activated shifts as the point (or the image) in the visual field shifts. The presence of a block of tissue representing a point in visual space reflects the rather coarse detail of this map. Consequently, two electrode penetrations would have to be spaced very far apart for them to locate neurons whose receptive fields did not share common points in visual space.

The deep-layer map is not only coarser than the superficial one, but includes an area of visual space rarely represented in superficial-layer neurons: the far periphery. The deep-layer map encompasses the entire contralateral visual field and also extends farther into ipsilateral space than does the superficial map. As depicted in figure 6.2, ipsilateral and central visual space occupy the rostral and rostrolateral aspects of the

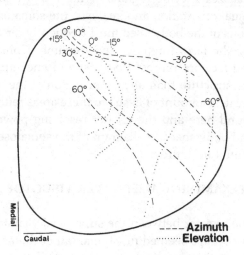

Figure 6.2 Visual map in deep layers of cat. Note that despite differences from the superficial-layer map, the orientations of the meridians are quite similar. The dotted 0° line represents the horizontal meridian (it has 0° of elevation), and runs rostral-caudal. The dashed 0° line represents the vertical meridian (it has 0° of azimuth), and runs medial-lateral. Minus and plus signs refer to inferior and superior visual space, respectively.

deep layers, while temporal visual space is found caudally; points superior or inferior are represented medially or laterally. Despite the coarser and more extensive visuotopy in deep layers, the overall pattern with which visual space is represented is similar to that found superficially, and the two visuotopies are in closest alignment in their representations of central visual space.

SOMATOSENSORY REPRESENTATION

Like their visual counterparts, somatosensory neurons have large receptive fields and are organized into a somatotopic map. The somatotopy was first documented long before a deep-layer visual map had been determined, and at the time, the well-defined superficial visuotopy appeared to be an excellent reference for seeking the organizational pattern of the body representation. This was done by recording along long vertical electrode penetrations extending from the surface of the superior colliculus to the underlying tegmentum (Stein et al. 1976b). Visual receptive fields were mapped superficially in each electrode penetration, and the somatosensory receptive fields found in the deep layers were then related to the centers of the overlying visual receptive fields in the same electrode penetrations. A very regular relationship between the visual map and the somatotopic map was found. Regions of the deep layers representing the face were found lying under visual receptive fields representing the area centralis, forelimb was found beneath inferior temporal visual fields, and trunk and hindlimb were beneath far temporal visual receptive fields. Just as the visual map emphasizes specific regions of the retina that are used most heavily for visual orientation and analysis, the somatosensory map emphasizes regions of the body used most frequently for tactile orientation and analysis: the face, forepaw, and forelimb. Consequently, the central retina and face are represented best and encompass proportionately more of the structure than any other region of the retina or body. Devoting the greatest amount of tissue to these areas reflects the small receptive fields found here and the greater resolving power in these regions of visual and body space. A diagram of the somatosensory representation is presented in figure 6.3A.

REEXAMINING DEEP-LAYER VISUOTOPY AND SOMATOTOPY

The register between the superficial visuotopic and deep-layer somatotopic maps seemed functional rather than coincidental. For example, an object that approached and touched the left side of the animal's face would lead to coincident activation of somatosensory and visual inputs, producing a vertical column of activity extending through all layers. Funneling this activity to a limited focus within the deep layers in this way seemed to be a particularly effective way of maximally activating a

Multiple, Overlapping Sensory and Motor Maps

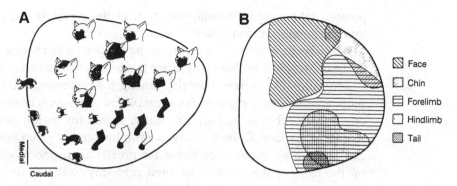

Figure 6.3 Body map. Whether using standard receptive field mapping techniques (*A*, from Stein et al. 1976b) or quantitative evaluative methods (*B*, from Meredith et al. 1991), similar deep-layer maps of the body surface are evident: the front of the animal is represented rostral while its hindparts are caudal; the upper surface of the animal is represented medial and its lower aspects lateral.

localized group of deep-layer efferent neurons. This, in turn, would maximize the likelihood of a properly directed orientation.

Conceptually linking visual and somatosensory function in this way assumed that there is an intimate interaction among superficial visual neurons and deep somatosensory and output neurons; however, there is no evidence that such an association exists (indeed, there is no evidence that superficial visual neurons can influence deep layer nonvisual, multisensory, or output neurons). The fact that the visual maps in the superficial and deep layers are roughly aligned allows the logic of hypotheses based on the presence of visual-nonvisual registry to be retained. Only now, the visual map used as a referent is restricted to the deep layers. Just why the superficial and deep layers, with their different afferent patterns and behavioral involvements, have visual maps that are so well aligned remains unclear, but recent findings that there are connections between superficial and deep-layer visual neurons (see chapter 3) indicate that superficial neurons might contribute to behaviors mediated by the deep layers in ways we do not yet understand.

Reexamining the somatosensory representation with the point-image technique used to study the deep-layer visual map reveals a number of fundamental similarities between them. The organization of the somatotopic map remains basically the same as previously described, but it becomes evident that the somatotopy, like the deep-layer visuotopy, is better described as a blocklike pattern than as a point-to-point organization (Meredith et al. 1991). Its general scheme is shown in figure 6.3B and can be compared to that shown in figure 6.3A. The head has the largest representation, occupying nearly the entire rostral half of the structure, and the map is oriented so that the scalp is medial to the chin. The second largest representation is devoted to the forelimb, localized primarily to the lateral aspects of the caudal two thirds of the structure. The remainder of the body (the trunk, belly, hindlimb, and tail) is compressed into a region overlapping part of the forelimb and extending into the small remaining caudal zone.

While regions of the body surface have specific territories or blocks of tissue devoted to them, these are by no means exclusive, and there is a considerable degree of overlap among the representations of one or more adjacent body regions. For example, neurons with receptive fields on the forelimb may be found rostrally, within the region devoted primarily to the face. Consequently, a stimulus on any given body region can activate an expanse of tissue far greater than one would predict on the basis of the territory devoted primarily to that body part. This widespread activation might help increase the likelihood of detecting an event simply by activating many neurons, but if (as is generally assumed) locating the position of the stimulus depends on limiting the focus of activity in the structure, this organization will also appear to produce some problems (see chapter 12).

AUDITORY REPRESENTATION

It might now be assumed that since the visual and somatosensory representations are arranged in maplike patterns, the auditory representation should follow suit. This assumption is not nearly as straightforward as it might seem. In both the visual and somatosensory systems each peripheral nerve fiber responds to a stimulus in a restricted (generally contralateral) spatial domain, regardless of stimulus intensity, and this defines the cell's receptive field. Consequently, it is comparatively easy to understand how the central nervous system constructs a spatial map of the contralateral visual field and the contralateral body surface. In contrast, each primary auditory nerve fiber can respond to a loud sound regardless of its location in space—there is no spatial map at the peripheral receptor, and the auditory system is organized at both thalamic and cortical levels according to sound frequencies, or tones (i.e., *tonotopic*), and not according to auditory space (*spatiotopic*). Therefore, the construction of a spatial auditory map in the superior colliculus would have to be the result of a computation based on the differences in the intensity and timing of sound as it reaches the two ears. This is, in fact, how such a map is accomplished.

Sensitivity to interaural time and intensity differences are the principal response features of superior colliculus neurons. Coupled with the physical features of the external ear that aid in sound localization (Palmer and King 1985), these interaural properties are the basis for the auditory receptive fields that have been observed repeatedly in the superior colliculus (Gordon 1973; Harris et al. 1980; King and Palmer 1983, 1985; Palmer and King 1983, 1985; Middlebrooks and Knudsen 1984; Meredith and Stein 1986b; Middlebrooks 1987). When one examines the most responsive, or best, areas of the receptive fields of auditory neurons, a spatiotopic map of auditory space becomes evident

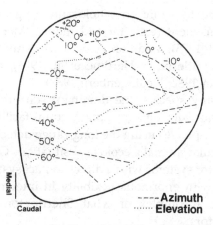

Figure 6.4 Auditory space map. Positions of increasing azimuth (from nasal to temporal) are represented rostral to caudal (dashed lines), while increasing elevations (dotted lines, from inferior to superior) are represented medial to lateral. (Modified from Middlebrooks and Knudsen 1984. Reprinted by permission of the *Journal of Neuroscience*)

(Middlebrooks and Knudsen 1984). This computational map is oriented very much like the visual and somatosensory maps, indicating that the same axes are used to represent all three sensory modalities. Thus, the auditory horizontal meridian is laid out rostral-caudally across the structure and its vertical meridian is laid out medial-laterally, as shown in figure 6.4, providing a reasonably good parallel to the visual and somatosensory representations.

SIMILAR VISUAL AND NONVISUAL MAPS IN OTHER MAMMALS

Although the details presented above are drawn from data gathered in the cat, a general correspondence of visual and nonvisual maps has been observed in other laboratory mammals, including rat (McHaffie et al. 1989), hamster (Tiao and Blakemore 1976; Chalupa and Rhoades 1977; Finlay et al. 1978; Stein and Dixon 1979; Larson et al. 1987), mouse (Drager and Hubel 1975), guinea pig (King and Palmer 1983), rabbit (Schaefer 1970), and ferret (King and Hutchins 1987). It is also consistent with what is known about primates (Cynader and Berman 1972; Goldberg and Wurtz 1972a,b). This is not to say that the sensory representations in one species are the same as those in any other. Quite the contrary. What remains constant across species is not necessarily the specifics of a given set of sensory maps, but rather the general plan of overlapping the different sensory representations. Species vary considerably in the sensory modalities they depend on most for exploring and responding to environmental stimuli, and the neuron types represented in their superior colliculi faithfully reflect these dependencies. The sensory representations in primates and carnivores, which make heavy use of vision, contrast sharply with those in the midbrain of species that depend far more on echolocation (e.g., bat: Jen et al. 1984), whisker displacement (e.g., rat and mouse: McHaffie et al. 1989; Drager and Hubel 1975), audition (e.g., owl: Knudsen 1982), infrared detection (e.g., rattlesnake: Hartline et al. 1978), or electroreception (e.g., fish: Bastian 1982; Heilingenberg 1988).

In any species, the dominant sensory modality represented in the superior colliculus (or optic tectum) facilitates the initiation of anticipatory responses using the long-range detectors that are best suited to that particular animal's ecological situation. Coupling two or more distance receptor systems with a direct contact system, like skin, provides organisms with enormous flexibility in interacting with their environments using a complex of what Sherrington (1906/1947) called "externo-receptors."

Particularly interesting is the elaborate adaptation of a direct contact system in rodents: the whiskers, or vibrissae. Unlike primates or many other large mammals, rodents depend on their whiskers for a host of locomotor behaviors (Vincent 1912). Oddly enough, the loss of the whiskers produces disadvantages even in behaviors that on first consideration seem not to require their use, such as fighting and swimming. The extensive use of their whiskers for attentive and orientation functions is reflected in the abundance of neurons in their superior colliculi activated by whisker stimulation (Drager and Hubel 1975; McHaffie and Stein 1981; Rhoades et al. 1987; McHaffie et al. 1989; Kao et al. 1989, 1990). The whisker representation is also in rough spatial register with the visual map; the organization of the whisker representation is shown in figure 6.5.

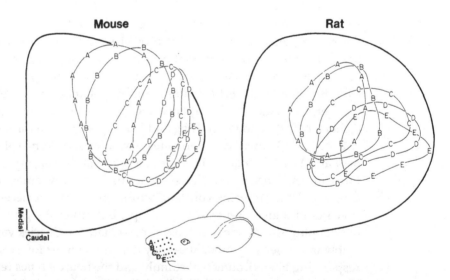

Figure 6.5 The whisker representation in rodent. The rows of whiskers, A through E (from dorsal to ventral), are represented (from medial to lateral) primarily in the rostral-lateral quadrant of the superior colliculus. (Modified from Drager and Hubel 1975 [mouse], and Kao et al. 1989 [rat])

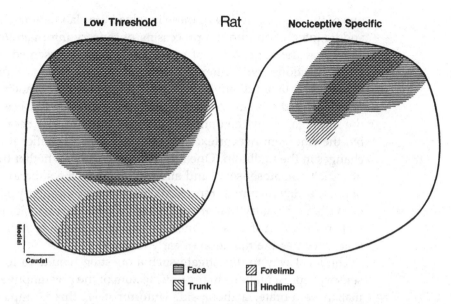

Figure 6.6 Low-threshold versus nociceptive-specific map in rat. Neurons sensitive to low-intensity somatic stimuli are found on all regions of the body and are distributed across the structure in somatotopic fashion. The receptive fields of neurons responsive only to noxious stimuli are not found in all body regions. Rather, they are restricted to the face and forelimb, and their distribution is limited to the rostral aspects of the superior colliculus. (From McHaffie et al. 1989)

By depending so extensively on the whiskers, the rodent puts its face at great risk during normal exploratory behavior. One recent postulate holds that the rodent's face (and its representation in the superior colliculus) is well adapted for exploration because the exquisitely sensitive whisker-activated system used for orientation and approach evolved in concert with a nociceptive-activated system for withdrawal (McHaffie et al. 1989). Since both reactions must be related to the location of the initiating stimulus on the body, neurons responsive to innocuous cues and those responsive to noxious stimuli have overlapping maps in the superior colliculus (figure 6.6). Once again, the preeminence of the plan of overlapping sensory maps is obvious despite striking variations in the physiology of the constituent neurons. Although neurons with similar receptive field and/or response properties may sometimes be found in clusters, a neuron's location in the superior colliculus is specified principally by its activating region in sensory space and not by submodality specialization.

PRINCIPLES OF SENSORY REPRESENTATIONS AND THE EVOLUTION AND RADIATION OF EARLY MAMMALS

During the evolutionary transition from reptilian to mammalian forms, a host of changes in brain organization took place. As discussed earlier, one of the most profound of these involved the elaboration of neocortex and its integration into the processing of sensory information. It is unlikely that the appearance of neocortex simply represented an adding on of functions, but rather a significant reorganization of preexisting networks to take full advantage of the higher-order capabilities of this new part of the brain. A common assumption is that at least some of the roles played by the optic tectum were shifted to, or became shared by, the emergent neocortex. This would result in significant functional changes in the midbrain. One might wonder, then, whether the register of visual, somatosensory, and auditory maps in the superior colliculus of present-day mammals represents one of the evolutionary adaptations of midbrain circuitry that arose during the period of transition to mammalian forms, or if it is an ancient scheme of modality representation that antedates the radiation of early mammals.

The ideal way to investigate such a question would be to detail the sensory representations in the optic tectum of the presumptive premammalian vertebrate, a therapsid. Unfortunately, this is impossible, for these mammal-like reptiles have been extinct for about as long as mammals have been extant. Consequently, the organizational commonalities must be compared in species that have diverged from the same extinct ancestor in order to test hypotheses about the origin of these overlapping sensory maps. This prompted us (Gaither and Stein 1979; Stein and Gaither 1981, 1983) to examine the optic tectum of the lizard *Iguana iguana*, since both lizards and mammals are believed to have evolved from the same primitive stem-reptiles (Romer 1970).

Reptiles

The optic tectum of the iguana was studied in much the same way as was the superior colliculus in cat and rodent, and a well-organized visual map was found. It was composed of very small, discrete receptive fields. Many of these neurons had properties quite similar to those detailed in mammals (Stein and Gaither 1983), and despite a rotation of the horizontal and vertical meridians, the visuotopy looked very much like that found in cat—it even included a similar magnification of the central visual field (Stein and Gaither 1981). As in cat, deeper-layer visual neurons in the iguana had larger receptive fields than those found superficially, and many somatosensory and bimodal neurons were found in the deep layers. Regardless of whether one compares unimodal visual and unimodal somatosensory receptive fields or the receptive fields of multisensory neurons, a close spatial correspondence of the different sensory maps is apparent. The visuotopic-somatotopic maps and their registry found in the iguana are summarized in figure 6.7.

Reptiles living in very different environments and with far more exotic detection apparatus than those of the iguana also exhibit a close

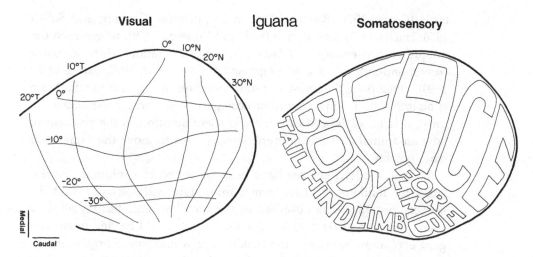

Figure 6.7 Visual and body representations in the reptilian optic tectum. Maps of the visual field and body in the iguana optic tectum are in register with one another: nasal (N) and central visual space corresponds to the representation of the face, temporal (T) visual space corresponds to the trunk and caudal body parts, and inferior visual space is in register with inferior body parts. (Modified from Stein and Gaither 1981)

spatial registration of sensory representations in their optic tecta. A particularly elegant demonstration of this has been provided by Hartline and associates (1978) in rattlesnake. The rattlesnake, like other pit vipers, possesses a pair of infrared organs (i.e., pits), one on each side of the face (Terashima and Goris 1975), which it uses quite effectively to direct strikes at warm objects. The infrared organ's view of the world is represented in maplike form in the optic tectum and is in spatial register with the superficial visual representation (except at caudal sites, which represent the far peripheral field). These observations indicate that the rule of intersensory spatial register is not limited to a specific set of externoreceptors.

Birds, Amphibians, and Fish

Birds have sometimes been called "flying reptiles" because of the many similarities they have to their progenitors. These similarities are not restricted to physiognomy, but extend to the organization of the central nervous system and especially to the presence of spatiotopic sensory representations in their optic tecta. Perhaps nowhere is this more evident than in the common barn owl, an extremely effective nighttime hunter with an uncanny sense of hearing. Compared to the superior colliculi or optic tecta of visually dominant species, the optic tectum of the owl is very heavily devoted to its auditory representation. But it, too, shows the same sort of visual-auditory spatial register as in mammals and reptiles (Knudsen 1982). A general correspondence between sensory representations in the midbrain also has been reported in other birds (Cotter 1976; Ballam 1982), in amphibians (Gruberg and Solish 1978; Harris 1982), and in fish (Fish and Voneida 1979), where even the unique electrosensory and lateral line representations show a coarse correspondence to the visual representation (Bastian 1982; Bartels et al. 1990). Obviously, the register of sensory representations in the midbrain is adaptive in a wide variety of ecological situations, presumably because it is an early and extremely efficient solution to the problem of how an animal can use different sensory cues to move the same body parts quickly.

Because modern species have been subjected to evolutionary pressures for millions of years, one cannot state with certainty that the sensory organizations observed in the reptilian optic tectum reflect a premammalian characteristic. The similarities could be due to convergent evolution. However, the striking similarities in the organizational features of the sensory maps in the optic tecta and superior colliculi of widely divergent species living in very different ecological situations make it far more likely that an ancestral plan was retained during the emergence of mammals more than 180 million years ago. The species-specific differences that do exist today appear to reflect modifications of this common plan rather than its repeated, independent discovery by each new group of animals. The fact that the fundamental features of sensory represention in the midbrain are present in amphibians and fish suggests that the roots of this plan lie even further back in vertebrate evolution than the stem-reptile.

7 Motor Maps

The primary role of the superior colliculus is to translate a sensory stimulus into a signal that will produce an appropriate orientation of the peripheral sensory organs. To accomplish this there is neuronal specialization within the structure. Some neurons are devoted to processing sensory inputs, others to organizing motor responses, while many others have dual roles, both sensory and motor. Ultimately, activation of superior colliculus neurons orients (or in some cases protects) the very organs from which the structure derives its sensory information (i.e., eyes, ears, head and body). This centers the stimulus with respect to the animal, who is now in the best position to interact with it and to analyze its characteristics in detail (see figure II.1). Although referred to as *premotor* (or sometimes as *motor*), the effector, or efferent, neurons of the superior colliculus accomplish their role polysynaptically through widespread connections with neurons in other motor areas of the brain stem and spinal cord, as shown schematically in figure 3.3. But these schematics give little clue to the well-organized maps on which these motor connections must be based, an organization that is immediately apparent from studies using electrical stimulation techniques.

EYE MOVEMENTS

The ubiquitous nature of overlapping sensory and motor maps is apparent from microstimulation studies in many species. An electrical stimulus presented in, for example, a site representing superior temporal visual space will move the eyes superiorly and temporally, as if to center the fovea (or its equivalent) on the visual location represented at the stimulation site (Syka and Radil-Weiss 1971; Robinson 1972; Schiller and Stryker 1972; Stein et al. 1976a; McHaffie and Stein 1982). Although, as noted earlier, the "foveation" hypothesis offered to explain the function and organization of these movements has been modified to emphasize a motor coordinate rather than a retinocentric system (Sparks and Mays 1983), and to take into account observations that both eye and head movements are involved in the redirection of gaze (Munoz and Guitton 1989; Harris 1980) (see the earlier discussion of the premotor neurons

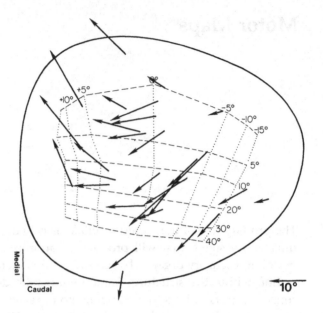

Figure 7.1 Eye movement map. The direction and amplitude of electrical stimulation-induced eye movements depend on the site of stimulation and are in general register with the visual map: stimulation of the medial aspect of the structure, where the upper visual field is represented, elicits upward eye movements, while more lateral stimulation, in the area of the representation of the inferior visual field, evokes downward eye movements. The length and angle of each arrow indicate the amplitude and direction of the evoked eye movement. (Redrawn from McIlwain 1990)

involved in these behaviors in chapter 4), the point regarding sensory and oculomotor register remains clearly evident: they overlap one another within the animal's oculomotor range. Therefore, the representation of a region of sensory space and the representation of the signals required to move the eyes toward that region are in the same superior colliculus location (figure 7.1).

Because the sensory and motor maps covary, during any shift of gaze a dynamic change in activity must take place across the superior colliculus. As noted in chapter 2, this has been postulated in a recent study by Munoz and co-workers (1991) and can stand reiteration in the present context. During visual fixation, neurons in the rostral aspect of the superior colliculus are active, apparently holding the eyes in fixation. These fixation neurons become quiet when gaze is to be redirected, for example, to a far peripheral visual target. To initiate the movement to the far periphery, premotor activity occurs in the caudal superior colliculus, where far peripheral visual space is represented. According to their hypothesis then, the zone of activity must sweep rostrally across the structure as gaze is shifted toward the target, with the zone of activity at any given point during the excursion reflecting the remaining gaze error. Once the new target is fixated, the site of activity is once again in the rostral superior colliculus. Although there are no comparable data for premotor ear movement activity, an ear movement map has also been demonstrated in cat superior colliculus (Stein and Clamann 1981).

EAR MOVEMENTS

Stein and Clamann (1981) used the same preparation for studying eye movements to reveal a well-ordered ear movement map in the cat superior colliculus. One can use the auditory map to predict electrically evoked ear movements if one simply assumes that the stimulus mimics the effect of a sound, and that the ear movements function to "fixate" that sound. Consequently, stimulation of rostral sites produces forward movements of the contralateral ear, stimulation of caudal sites produces backward movements, medial sites produce upward movements and lateral sites produce downward movements (figure 7.2). The ear ipsilateral to the stimulated superior colliculus moves in synchrony, so that the effect of mimicking an auditory stimulus slightly to the left and below the head results in both ears moving toward the left and down. If the presumptive sound is far to the left, so that ready access to the right ear (the ear ipsilateral to the relevant superior colliculus) is blocked by the head, the right ear does not move at all. This ear movement map is quite similar to the eye movement map and, as shown in figure 7.2,

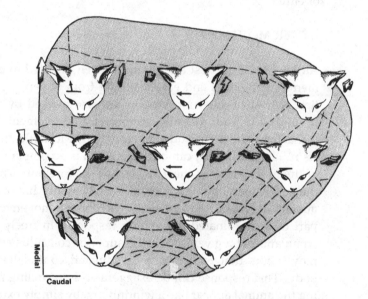

Figure 7.2 Eye and ear movement maps are in register. Electrical stimulation produces movements of the ears (from dotted position to shaded), and eyes (small arrows) toward the contralateral sensory field. The large arrows indicate the relative amplitude and direction of the evoked ear movements in these head-fixed animals. Note the parallel movements: stimulation of medial sites evokes eye and ear movements with strong upward components, while lateral stimulation produces downward movements; stimulation of rostral sites produces relatively small movements, while caudal-most stimulation sites elicit large movements (in this case only the contralateral ear moved). (Redrawn from Stein and Clamann 1981)

microstimulation at any point in deep superior colliculus evokes conjugate movements of the eyes and the ears. These movements are accomplished via polysynaptic superior colliculus connections to the ear muscles (Vidal et al. 1988).

The rabbit is arguably a more auditory animal than is the cat. Its large mobile ears sit near the top of the head so that auditory stimuli are largely unobstructed. In keeping with the rabbit's extensive use of auditory cues, ear movements are more readily evoked from its superior colliculus than are eye movements—the opposite of that in the cat. Furthermore, the eyes are located more lateral in the head in rabbit and there is a much greater proportion of crossed retinal input (and less binocularity) than found in the cat. Therefore, each superior colliculus contains a larger field of view of the contralateral side of the animal. Yet despite these obvious differences in visual and auditory organization, there is an ear movement map in the rabbit superior colliculus that is aligned with its eye movement map (Schaefer 1970), just as is found in the cat.

Obviously, motor maps, like sensory maps, will have many species-specific features, but it would be as surprising to find motor maps unaligned with one another in any species as it would be to find sensory maps unaligned with one another. Thus far there have been no reports of either.

OTHER MOVEMENTS

Although the greatest attention has been devoted to orientation movements of the eyes and ears resulting from superior colliculus stimulation, a host of other movements are also evoked by such stimulation. In both cat and rodents, contralateral movement of the whiskers (Schaefer 1970; Stein and Clamann 1981; McHaffie and Stein 1982; see also Vidal et al. 1988) can be evoked and is accompanied by movements of the mouth and/or cheek as well as the forelimb. The organization of these whisker, mouth, and limb movements has not yet been adequately described; nevertheless, each of the movements appears to be part of a coordinated orientation response. In freely moving animals, stimulation at a given site in the superior colliculus evokes a concert of movements that results in a coordinated contralateral turning of the body. This response can be exaggerated into circling movements, making the animal appear like a windup toy, by simply extending the period of stimulation.

If the electrical current presented at some sites in the superior colliculus is of sufficiently high frequency or intensity, it may provoke the opposite reactions: withdrawal or escape. This has been demonstrated most clearly in rodents. As noted earlier, there is good reason to suspect that this reflects the involvement of the superior colliculus in withdrawal from potentially damaging noxious stimuli. However, there is also reason to suspect that innocuous stimuli (e.g., a looming visual stimulus) that signal danger may also evoke withdrawal movements via the circuitry of the superior colliculus (Westby et al. 1990), but it is not yet clear whether the specific overt movements that are evoked by noxious stimuli and looming visual stimuli exhibit an overall register (or "antiregister") with the nociceptive and/or visual maps.

MOTOR MAPS IN NONMAMMALIAN SPECIES

Compared to the data available on the premotor properties of superior colliculus neurons in mammals and the detailed maps of electrically evoked eye, ear, and gaze movements in these animals, the information on the motor representations in the optic tectum of nonmammalian species seems somewhat sparse. Nevertheless, there is good reason to believe that analogous motor organizations existed in the midbrain long before the advent of mammals. Bullock (1984) summarizes the results of a number of studies done in the late 1920s and the early 1930s in which the effects of electrical stimulation in the rays *Trygon* and *Myliobatis* were examined. Rays are very ancient species of cartilaginous fish that show evidence of a crude motor topography in their optic tecta (although Bullock notes that these particular studies need confirmation). Stimulation of the lateral tectum produced movements of the ipsilateral wing, whereas stimulation of the medial tectum produced movements of the contralateral wing. Stimulation at successive points along the rostrocaudal axis of the tectum produced the same series of movements of the ipsilateral wing (when stimulation was lateral) and the contralateral wing (when stimulation was medial): rostral stimulation produced movements of the anterior portion of the wing, middle stimulation produced movements of the middle of the wing, and caudal stimulation produced movements of the posterior portion of the wing. Well-organized electrically evoked eye and body movements have also been demonstrated in teleost fishes (Vanegas et al. 1984).

The studies in the optic tecta of the freely moving lizard and salamander are more directly comparable to mammals. Electrical stimulation of the optic tectum in the iguana produces orientation movements that bring the eye to view the approximate region of the visual field represented at the stimulation site (Stein and Gaither 1981), as shown in figure 7.3. This is quite similar to the results of electrical stimulation of the superior colliculus in freely moving mammals. Furthermore, the orientation movements evoked from the optic tectum are stereotyped and yet are quite similar to the avoidance movements elicited when the experimenter's hand approaches the animal from one side or the other.

Particularly provocative are the evoked movements that have been reported in salamander. Finkenstadt and Ewert (1983) showed not only that electrically evoked orientation movements in the salamander correspond to the retinotectal map (as they do in mammals), but that a com-

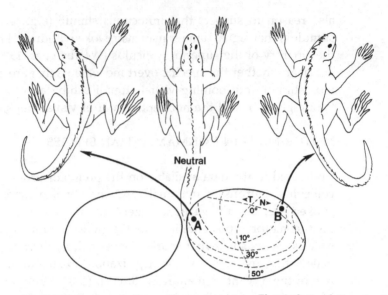

Figure 7.3 Orientation map in the reptilian optic tectum. Electrical stimulation at a site in the right optic tectum that represents temporal visual space (A) produces a contralateral (temporal, T) turning of the head toward the presumptive stimulus, while stimulation at a site representing nasal visual space (B) elicits an ipsilateral (nasal, N) turning movement. Isobars of the visual field are plotted in polar coordinates on the schematic of the optic tectum. Note that the orientation of the visual map is shifted approximately 90° from that in the mammal. (From Stein and Gaither 1981)

plex series of movements can be evoked in these animals consisting of orientation, stalking, snapping, and biting. This series of electrically evoked movements bears a striking similarity to the animal's normal prey-catching behaviors. In some cases avoidance movements could also be evoked. Similarly, components of prey-capturing behaviors can be elicited from the optic tecta and the subjacent tegmentum in frogs and toads, which possess a "snapping" area (Comer and Grobstein 1981; Ewert 1984; Satou et al. 1985).

Although approach, avoidance, and even movements of the mouth are evoked by electrical stimulation of the mammalian superior colliculus, the well-organized predation-like behaviors that are evoked from the amphibian optic tectum do not have an obvious parallel among mammals. The motor patterns represented in the optic tectum appear to be composed of much more involved behavioral sequences than those represented in the superior colliculus; they have the appearance of complete behaviors that are indistinguishable from those evoked by natural stimuli. Perhaps this difference between mammals and nonmammals reflects a redistribution of the components of complex behavioral repertoires in species with a well-developed neocortex. Thus, the bird, whose cortex has developed far beyond its reptilian ancestors, shows a tectal motor organization quite similar to that of the mammal. The owl has essentially no independent eye movement control, but its head-movement map in the tectum is comparable to the eye- or gaze-control map in the superior colliculus (Du Lac and Knudsen 1990).

Despite species-specific differences, the midbrain of every species studied, from ancient fishes to modern mammals, contains well-organized sensory and motor maps that are in register with one another. These observations lend support to the notion that both sensory overlap and sensory-motor overlap are ancient schemes of midbrain organization that were likely to have been retained in the evolutionary transition from reptilian to mammalian species because they are useful in a wide variety of ecological situations. As will be shown in the remainder of this volume, this provides a mechanism for integrating the information contained in the sensory messages of different modalities and for giving the different senses access to the same midbrain-mediated behaviors.

IV Multisensory Convergence and Integration at the Level of the Single Neuron

Our studies of multisensory integration arose directly from the investigations of unimodal sensory processing in the cat superior colliculus that were described in part III. Over the years a number of unsystematic observations accumulated indicating that the properties of the multisensory neurons that were encountered were far more complicated than we had first imagined on the basis of their responses to modality-specific stimuli. An observation that immediately comes to mind occurred in an experiment with the late Steve Edwards to document the vertical distribution of different types of sensory neurons in the superior colliculus. We encountered a neuron that responded vigorously to a very-low-intensity auditory stimulus, and inadvertently noticed that it was completely suppressed when we covered the animal's eyes or turned all the room lights off so that it did not see the visual stimulus on the screen in front of it. It was quite late, the observation had nothing to do with this experiment, and we were eager to complete the experiment and go home. Still, the effect we noticed was so dramatic and so unexpected that we couldn't move on. In fact, we couldn't accept the obvious conclusion that the neuron would respond to an auditory stimulus only if there was some visual input at the same time. So the test was repeated 10 or 12 times with a variety of different auditory stimuli, but with the same results. After a while it became a game to find yet another auditory stimulus whose effect we could inhibit with darkness. This was interrupted by the inescapable late-night giddiness suffered (enjoyed?) by those who do electrophysiological experiments, and we finally concluded that cats must be deaf at night. This, of course, began a string of other ridiculous conclusions: blind cats are probably deaf too; and on and on.

As discussed in part I, there are many areas of the brains of many species in which multiple sensory afferents converge (figure IV.1). Presumably, any one of these areas could be useful in exploring the rules governing the integration of multiple sensory inputs. But for us the kind of example described above, in which two sensory stimuli could produce dramatic effects in the same superior colliculus neuron that would not be predicted from observing its reactions to either stimulus

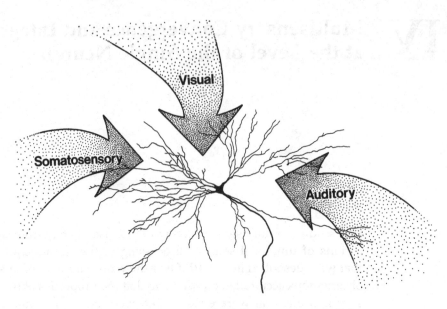

Figure IV.1 Convergence of inputs from the different senses on a single neuron.

alone, was compelling, and it made the cat superior colliculus seem a particularly apt structure for us to use to study interactions among sensory modalities. It also promised to help explain, at the cellular level, how two different sensory stimuli could function synergistically to enhance the detection of a stimulus. The superior colliculus has proved to be an exceptionally good choice, and the results of these experiments will be presented here in detail as a model of multisensory integration at the level of the single neuron. Hopefully, these studies presage additional data from a host of experiments in other structures and species that will extend these observations and help determine the general applicability of the model.

The maplike arrangements of sensory representations, coupled with the receptive field features of individual superior colliculus neurons discussed earlier, have been found to be key features in determining how different sensory inputs are integrated at the level of the single neuron. The heavy contribution of multisensory neurons to the organization of the different sensory maps indicates that there are integrated maps in the superior colliculus. This concept will be discussed in detail in chapter 8 and the effect of combining different sensory stimuli on the behavior of the multisensory neurons forming these maps will be examined in chapters 9–11. It is primarily the data base presented in chapters 9 and 10 that has led to the view that some reliable rules for the integration of information from different modalities exist in the superior colliculus, and may actually apply to other structures involved in other functions.

By the end of chapter 10 we should have made it clear that many of the most compelling inferences about multisensory integration drawn from neurophysiological and behavioral experiments are readily testable. Several predictions will then come to mind about what should happen (assuming that the rules of multisensory integration that we defined do not simply have face validity) if the substrate underlying these interactions is modified. Some of these predictions involve issues pertaining to the development (or lack thereof) of alignment among sensory maps when normal maturation is disrupted, and these will be dealt with in chapter 11. Others involve the consequences of perturbing the normal relationships among sensory modalities and/or receptive field properties, for if normal multisensory integration in the superior colliculus depends on the alignment of sensory representations and the normal complement of receptive field characteristics, altering either or both should result in a product that violates the rules of multisensory integration (as described here) or one that is maladaptive. Experimental approaches making use of this sort of strategy are still in their early stages; nevertheless, some initial findings are quite unexpected and have led to speculations that a radical revision of concepts of how the brain maintains sensory maps may be warranted. These observations and speculations, as well as some of the more immediate questions requiring appropriate experimental investigation, will be dealt with. Finally, the results of preliminary experiments with multisensory integration in two association areas of the cat brain, the anterior ectosylvian sulcus and the rostral portion of the lateral suprasylvian cortex, will be described. These data represent initial efforts to determine whether the same integrative effects observed in the superior colliculus are also present in other multisensory neurons.

8 Integrated Maps Formed by Multisensory Neurons

LARGE RECEPTIVE FIELDS, MULTISENSORY NEURONS, AND THE OVERLAP AMONG SENSORY REPRESENTATIONS

The use of common axes among the visual, auditory, and somatosensory representations in the superior colliculus allows a single composite diagram, as shown in figures 8.1 and 8.2, to describe them. The figures also help make it apparent how the auditory and somatosensory components of the multisensory representation can be described in visual coordinates and vice versa. Yet, despite the general alignment of the sensory representations, it should be recognized that great accuracy is not achieved in their spatial register; the large size of superior colliculus receptive fields appears to preclude it. This is most apparent among the different receptive fields of multisensory neurons. For example, it is quite rare to find a visual-auditory neuron whose two sensory receptive fields approach complete coincidence, and we have certainly never noticed the three receptive fields of a trimodal neuron to do so. When mapped on a common coordinate system, it becomes apparent that large portions of a multisensory neuron's receptive fields overlap, while others protrude from one another (figure 8.3). In terms of this overlap there does not appear to be any systematic plan for coupling different sensory receptive fields, and considerable variability occurs from neuron to neuron.

A possible advantage of this imprecision is that minor shifts of peripheral sensory organs are not very disruptive to the overall register among the representations, or among the different receptive fields of individual multisensory neurons. Small movements of one set of sensory organs will increase the degree of receptive field overlap in some neurons while simultaneously degrading it in others, yet the registry among the maps themselves remains largely intact. This ensures that stimuli of any modality in the same location in space activate neurons in the same region of the superior colliculus. However, large deviations of the eyes, ears, or body could produce significant problems of registry if there are not equivalent movements of the other peripheral sensory organs. Animals

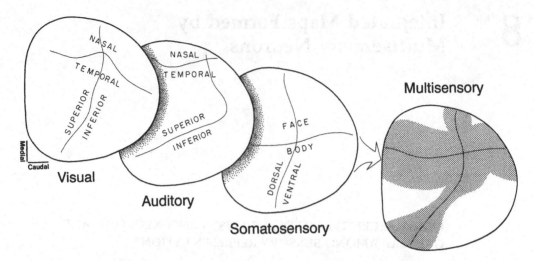

Figure 8.1 Visual-auditory-somatosensory correspondence in the superior colliculus. The horizontal and vertical meridians of the different sensory representations in the superior colliculus are quite similar. This common coordinate system suggests a representation of "multisensory space," as shown in figure 8.2.

are clearly capable of making such large and selective movements of individual sensory organs and often do so. Possible strategies for dealing with this situation are discussed in chapter 12.

It is likely that the use of similar spatial schemes to represent each sensory modality in the superior colliculus is the most economical way of specifying the location of peripheral stimuli, and of organizing and activating the motor program required to orient to them. But because the various sensory representations in deep superior colliculus have large receptive fields which are not organized in the typical point-to-point manner, even small stimuli will activate many neurons over a wide block of tissue. As a consequence, the activity of an individual neuron, and even small groups of neurons, is ambiguous with regard to the precise location of the stimulus. Localization undoubtedly depends on the activation of a large enough pool of neurons to produce a concentrated pattern of activity that is easily differentiated from surrounding activity. A crude but effective image of the required sensory pattern is like that left on a target by a shotgun blast: a dense core and a speckled perimeter. The dense core and symmetrical perimeter will weight the activity of output neurons of the superior colliculus so that the proper orienting movement is initiated. The resolution of stimulus location is signaled not only by the distribution of active neurons, but also by differential levels of activity among these active neurons. The presence of "best areas" within receptive fields permits the same stimulus to evoke very different response magnitudes in neurons whose receptive fields occupy similar regions of the sensory field: it can fall within the best areas of some neurons and not others.

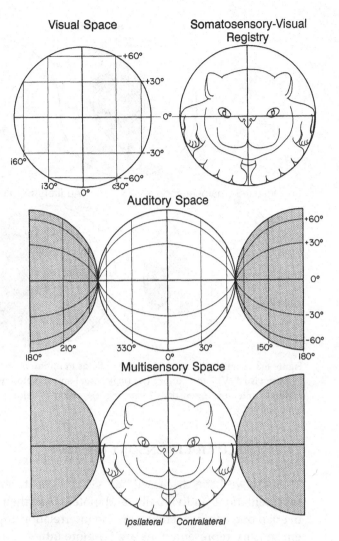

Figure 8.2 A multisensory spatial coordinate system. *Top left:* Visual space is depicted by a double-pole coordinate system with the intersection of the vertical and horizontal meridians (0° elevation, 0° azimuth) at the area centralis. Numbers with plus signs are in superior visual space, those with negative signs are in inferior visual space. *Top right:* The representation of the body in the superior colliculus as it would appear if mapped in visual coordinates. This map was constructed by plotting the body part at the center of the visual receptive field in each visual-somatosensory neuron sampled. For example, bimodal neurons with somatosensory receptive fields on the nose had visual receptive fields near the area centralis. *Center:* Auditory space shown in double-pole coordinates. Positions anterior to a line through the ears (the interaural axis) are depicted within the clear circle, while those posterior to it are represented by the darkened crescents on each side. These darkened crescents were detached from one another at the posterior midline (180°) and folded forward in order to flatten auditory space into a two-dimensional representation. *Bottom:* Auditory space is aligned with the overlapping visual and somatosensory representations (*upper right*) to produce a schematic of multisensory space (also see figure 8.1).

Integrated Maps Formed by Multisensory Neurons

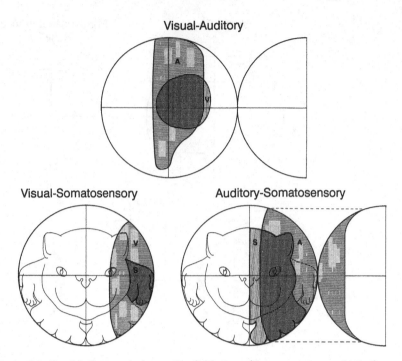

Figure 8.3 Spatial alignment of receptive fields in multisensory neurons. Note the overlapping visual (V) and auditory (A) (*top*); visual and somatosensory (S) (*bottom left*); and auditory and somatosensory (*bottom right*) receptive fields in three typical bimodal neurons.

INTEGRATED MULTISENSORY MAP(S)

Thus far we have discussed the visual, somatosensory, and auditory representations individually and noted that their maps parallel and overlap one another. However, the interrelationships among the different sensory representations are far more intimate than a simple parallel among individual organizations may indicate. Because the largest group of sensory neurons in the deep layers of the cat superior colliculus is multisensory (see chapter 9), an effective sensory stimulus, regardless of its modality, activates many of the same neurons, thereby enhancing its salience. This was quite evident when examining the individual sensory maps. Visual-multisensory neurons are not clustered in one region of the superior colliculus representing one region of visual space. Rather, they cover the entire structure so that the overwhelming majority of neurons from which the visual map (see figure 6.2) is constructed are multisensory, and this proves to be true for the somatosensory map (see figure 6.3) as well. At the moment, there is no reason to doubt that the same is also true of the auditory map. Presumably, the use of the same neurons to construct different sensory maps is not peculiar to certain mammals, but is a fundamental vertebrate characteristic.

Since the different sensory maps in the superior colliculus are composed of many of the same neurons, it may be more appropriate to think of them as components of a supramodal, or integrated, multisensory map (or as interlinked multisensory maps), rather than as three remarkably parallel but independent maps. It may, in fact, be the development of a register of receptive fields within individual bimodal and trimodal neurons that is the primary factor producing the maps' covariance. Despite the economy of the concept of integrated sensory maps for evaluating the functional organization of the superior colliculus, the possible roles of unimodal neurons should not be minimized. It appears that the integrated multisensory maps that allow different sensory modalities to gain access to the same circuits coexist with unimodal maps that preserve modality-specific access to output circuits.

AN INTEGRATED MULTISENSORY-MULTIMOTOR MAP?

The data discussed in the last section illustrate that there is a general register among sensory and motor maps. Because the notion is both useful and conceptually simple, some of us have entertained the idea that all the sensory and motor maps are components of an integrated multisensory-multimotor map. Such an "integrated" map enables each sensory modality to produce a "multimotor" response, which consists of the coordinated movement of the eyes, ears, head, and body. Certainly the concept of an integrated sensory-motor map works well as a mnemonic device and as a useful theoretical construct in the design of research strategies. However, there is now good reason to believe that this is more than merely a convenient theoretical concept; it is likely to be a significant component of superior colliculus organization.

In order for the general concept of an integrated multisensory-multimotor "map" to be tenable, it is necessary only for stimuli originating from the same locations in sensory space to activate neighboring unimodal neurons (from different modalities) in the structure, and for these neurons to have access to at least one of the output targets that effect orientation. The "integration" in this case would reflect the coordination of multiple inputs and outputs at the same superior colliculus locus.

There is no reason to doubt that this is a fundamental component of superior colliculus organization. But the data also indicate that different modalities converge on the same neurons and that these same multisensory neurons ultimately influence different peripheral sensory organs. As already noted, the majority of descending output neurons are multisensory, and many have elaborate collaterals that project to multiple targets. Consequently, a stimulus that is seen, heard, or felt can activate the same neurons in the superior colliculus and these, in turn, can produce a coordinated series of premotor signals that ultimately initiates overt behavior. This is certainly the most parsimonious way to link the various inputs and outputs.

The available experimental evidence is consistent with the idea that at the same time that some sensory and premotor neurons process unimodal inputs independently via parallel circuits, a core of multisensory-multimotor neurons initiates movements via a common circuit. The advantage of the latter scheme is that it provides the opportunity to integrate different sensory inputs and to use the resultant supramodal signals to coordinate the movement of the different peripheral sensory organs. The profound changes in activity produced by converging inputs and the advantages of such a system for overt behaviors will be dealt with in detail in the following chapters.

It is now necessary to develop a more complete picture of the sensory and motor properties of the various tectofugal neurons based on their individual target structures. Undoubtedly there will be an unequal distribution of neuron types, ranging from unimodal neurons that have limited output targets to trimodal neurons that project to most or all of the targets structures of the superior colliculus. Determining the distribution of these neuron types, and how their very different response properties affect different target structures, is necessary before we can begin to understand how different circuits share or divide the sensorimotor roles of the structure. The ongoing studies designed to determine the output targets of unimodal and multisensory neurons discussed in previous chapters are a first step in this effort.

For the integrated signals of output neurons to be meaningful, it is essential that the different input modalities affect one another in systematic ways. Put another way, there must be consistent "rules" governing the nature of these interactions. It is reasonable to expect that these rules would be based on the specific inputs to a neuron that happen to be activated at any given time. Presumably, then, if the multisensory convergence pattern of a given neuron and the properties of its responses to unimodal stimuli were known, it might be possible to predict the kinds of interactions that would be evoked by combinations of stimuli. In part, this has proved to be true, as will be discussed in the following chapters.

9 Multisensory Convergence Patterns

ESTIMATES OF CONVERGENCE FREQUENCY VARY WITH
METHODS, AND CONVERGENCE PATTERNS VARY WITH SPECIES

The specific patterns with which different sensory inputs converge on superior colliculus neurons in cats have been sought in many studies; however, there is still some hesitation in stating categorically which modality combinations occur most frequently and in what percentages. The results seem to vary with the method of analysis used and the cleverness of the experimenters in finding the activating, or trigger, features for each of the neurons they study. Most commonly, these analyses have been based solely on the stimuli that evoke impulses from the neurons examined, and, although all subthreshold influences are ignored with this method, it has sometimes provided remarkably high estimates of multisensory convergence (e.g., 62%; Gordon 1973).

In our own analyses, we use a method that is far more sensitive to these subthreshold influences but, paradoxically, one that has not resulted in the highest estimates of multisensory convergence. However, this appears to be due to our estimates being based on all neurons encountered in the superior colliculus, including those unresponsive to sensory stimuli. The method involves quantitative evaluation of the effects of presenting two stimuli from different modalities (visual, auditory, somatosensory) independently as well as simultaneously in every neuron encountered; in this way even the non-impulse-generating influences of one stimulus (e.g., auditory) can be revealed by its modulation of the effects of another (e.g., visual).

Over half of all deep-layer neurons studied in this fashion proved to be influenced (either excited or inhibited) by stimuli from more than one sensory modality and were classified as multisensory. This figure was obtained even though "unresponsive" neurons were included in the sample (Meredith and Stein 1985, 1986a). Yet, despite the impressive proportion of multisensory neurons obtained, the figure is probably an underestimation of their actual percentage. Because every conceivable manipulation of each stimulus parameter within each modality could not possibly be accomplished with each neuron in these experiments,

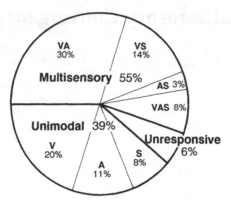

Figure 9.1 The patterns of sensory convergence in the superior colliculus.

one cannot exclude the possibility that a sensory input was present but not demonstrated. Furthermore, not all modalities were tested (e.g., noxious and vestibular stimuli were not presented). Nevertheless, despite the obvious caveats that such methodological limitations require, it is apparent that there is a representational hierarchy among the modalities examined (figure 9.1). Neurons with visual inputs predominate, and the most frequently encountered category is visual-auditory multisensory. This reflects the cat's heavy dependence on visual and auditory cues for orientation and contrasts sharply with that of other species. For example, somatosensory neurons abound in the rodent superior colliculus and the most frequent multisensory convergence pattern is visual-somatosensory (Drager and Hubel 1975; Weldon and Best 1992). This reflects the critical input from whiskers in these animals for orientation and object identification. Similarly, visual-infrared neurons are common in rattlesnake, an animal that makes extensive use of thermal cues to locate and capture warm-blooded prey (Hartline et al. 1978; Newman and Hartline 1981).

RECEPTIVE FIELD PROPERTIES DO NOT REFLECT MULTISENSORY CONVERGENCE PATTERNS

It might be expected that there are some special functional features of the neurons that receive multiple sensory inputs. One possibility is that only those neurons endowed with certain response properties will receive multiple sensory inputs and be able to participate in multisensory integration. So far, this appears not to be the case.

Except for a general increase in receptive field size as the number of converging modalities increases (i.e., unimodal receptive fields are smaller than bimodal receptive fields, which are smaller than trimodal receptive fields; Meredith et al. 1991), there is little to distinguish unimodal from bimodal or trimodal neurons: a visually responsive multisensory neuron is just as likely to be directionally selective, binocular, and to show spatial summation (or any other visual property) as is a unimodal visual neuron. Apparently, the sensory convergence patterns that are determined early in life (Stein et al. 1973) have little influence over the organization of receptive field properties within individual modalities. Perhaps this is because the various projections to the superior colliculus are not segregated, by their physiological properties, according to whether they are destined for neurons that will remain unimodal or for neurons that will receive multiple inputs; they have an equal affinity for both. Consequently, unimodal and multisensory neurons have access to the same modality-specific information, appear to synthesize it in the same way, and therefore exhibit the same within-modality receptive field properties. However, it is not yet clear whether the convergence patterns that characterize the adult are already established at prenatal or early neonatal stages. It is not inconceivable that the adult patterns are "carved" from a more global initial pattern as a consequence of afferent activity. At this point we can be sure of only one factor that ultimately limits the patterns of converging afferents that survive to adulthood: topographic fidelity.

DOES MULTISENSORY CONVERGENCE TAKE PLACE AT THE DEEP-LAYER NEURON ITSELF?

Often there is an implicit assumption that multisensory convergence takes place at the superior colliculus neuron itself, and is not simply relayed from multisensory neurons elsewhere. In large part this assumption is derived from observations that the superior colliculus is innervated heavily by unimodal structures. However, a number of other observations also favor this interpretation, the first of which is the selective effects of cortical deactivation.

The sensory responses of superior colliculus neurons eventually come under the influence of cortex (Stein and Gallagher 1981), with each sensory cortex controlling responses to its modality-specific stimuli. Deactivating visual cortex by cooling it to a temperature at which cortical neurons become inactive has been shown to affect the visual responses of superior colliculus neurons (Wickelgren and Sterling 1969; Stein and Arigbede 1972; see also Hardy and Stein 1988), but not to have a general depressive effect on all types of superior colliculus activity, because auditory and somatosensory responses remain unchanged (Stein 1978). Similarly, deactivating somatosensory cortex affects somatosensory responses (Clemo and Stein 1986), and deactivating auditory cortex affects auditory responses (Meredith and Clemo 1989). These neurons were rarely tested to determine whether or not they were multisensory. However, in the few cases in which superior colliculus neurons were found to be multisensory in nature, eliminating the excitatory influences of

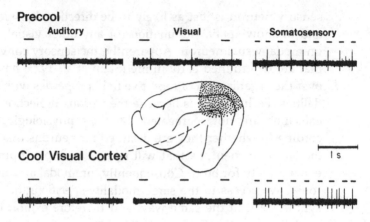

Figure 9.2 Deactivating visual cortex affects only visual responses in a multisensory neuron. Cooling visual cortex eliminated visual responses in this trimodal neuron, but auditory and somatosensory responses were unchanged. This suggests that the multisensory properties of this superior colliculus neuron are constructed from converging unimodal inputs. (Modified from Stein and Arigbede 1972)

visual cortex depressed their visual responses but had no effect on their somatosensory or auditory responses. An example of this modality selectivity is shown in figure 9.2.

The studies suggest that these corticotectal pathways are primarily unimodal; that their control over a multisensory neuron is limited to responses to a single sensory modality; and that different corticotectal pathways converge on the same neurons. To have confirmed these suggestions, however, the studies would have to have involved a more systematic examination of the reactions of the same multisensory superior colliculus neuron to deactivation of each of these different cortices. An ideal demonstration would be one in which the visual responses of a trimodal neuron are depressed by deactivating visual cortex, the somatosensory responses are depressed by deactivating somatosensory cortex, and the auditory responses are depressed by deactivating auditory cortex. Unfortunately, no such examples exist. Recently, however, we showed that electrical stimulation of lateral suprasylvian cortex, SIV, and Field AES can produce monosynaptic activation of the same superior colliculus neuron (figure 9.3) (Wallace et al. 1991). This is the best example we know showing direct convergence of different sensory inputs on the same superior colliculus neuron, and, taken together with previous observations, the data suggest that a good deal of multisensory convergence takes place directly on superior colliculus neurons. Furthermore, corticotectal neurons in those areas regarded as "polysensory association" areas are overwhelmingly (99%) unimodal (Wallace et al., unpublished observation). However, we cannot exclude the possibility that multisensory characteristics are assembled outside the superior colliculus, are relayed to it, and then are reflected in the properties of

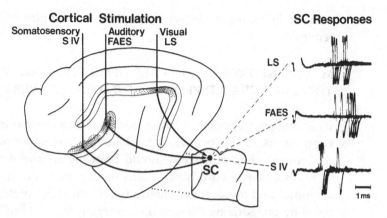

Cortical Stimulation

Somatosensory   Auditory   Visual
S IV   FAES   LS

SC Responses

LS

FAES

SC

S IV

1 ms

Figure 9.3 Multiple modality-specific cortices converge on superior colliculus neurons. Electrical stimulation of somatosensory (SIV), auditory (FAES), and visual (LS) cortices evokes orthodromic responses (*right*) in a trimodal superior colliculus neuron. The oscillograms represent the results of tests repeated six times for each area stimulated.

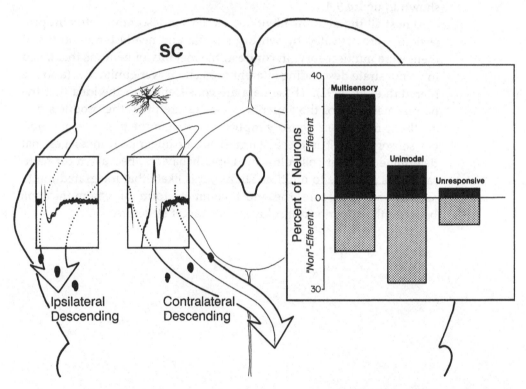

SC

Ipsilateral
Descending

Contralateral
Descending

Percent of Neurons

Efferent

"Non"-Efferent

40

0

30

Multisensory

Unimodal

Unresponsive

Figure 9.4 Multisensory neurons have descending efferent projections. Outputs from the superior colliculus reach brainstem and spinal cord targets through either ipsilateral or contralateral descending pathways (arrows). Stimulation was delivered through electrodes that straddled both pathways (electrode tips are represented by dark dots). The elicitation of antidromic spikes (insets on arrows) indicated that this neuron had an efferent projection in the contralateral descending pathway. The bar graph inset (*right*) shows that of the identified output neurons (dark bars), the majority were multisensory.

some of its neurons. As yet, however, no examples of this have been reported.

MULTISENSORY NEURONS ARE DESCENDING EFFERENTS AND THEIR INTEGRATED PRODUCT INFLUENCES OVERT BEHAVIOR

If, as suggested earlier, multisensory neurons are the most significant contributors to the behaviors mediated by the superior colliculus, its descending efferent system should be richly endowed with the axons of multisensory neurons. One can readily examine the proportion of unimodal and multisensory neurons projecting out of the superior colliculus by categorizing them and then trying to "backfire" them via antidromic stimulation of the two major descending output bundles. This was the technique we used to examine this question (Meredith and Stein 1985, 1986a; also see Guitton and Munoz 1991); the location of the tips of the stimulating electrodes relative to these efferent bundles is shown in figure 9.4.

Almost all the neurons identified as having descending efferent projections were activated by sensory stimuli, and nearly three-fourths of them were multisensory. In contrast, the majority of neurons that failed to demonstrate descending efferent projections were unimodal (also see Meredith et al. 1992). These data are consistent with the idea that the output messages of the superior colliculus are often the products of a synthesis of different sensory inputs, and that in the presence of different sensory cues it is these synthesized, or integrated, messages that determine superior colliculus–mediated behaviors. Because most natural events give rise to multiple stimuli, it is likely that integrated multisensory messages are the most common form of communication between the superior colliculus and its target structures.

10 Neural Consequences of Multisensory Interactions

Almost every environment contains an endlessly changing kaleidoscope of perceivable events, many of which are caused by the actions of the sensing beings themselves. Stimuli occur at various positions in space and time, and each animal must create perceptual order out of this seemingly bewildering array to produce an integrated, comprehensive assessment of its external world. In large part this is accomplished by attending to some complexes of stimuli and ignoring others. Obviously the process is successful only if an animal can determine which stimuli are related to one another and which are not. Since the individual sensory channels normally separate stimuli by modality without regard to the meaningfulness of stimulus combinations, to relate stimuli to one another the brain must reassemble relationships based on significance, not modality. Some of this assembling reflects the intrinsic circuitry of the brain, and some the product of postnatal experience as well. But in either case a similar mechanism is evident: certain combinations of stimuli become more salient because neuronal responses to them are enhanced, and other combinations of stimuli remain less salient (or become so) by producing the opposite effect, neuronal depression.

This sort of enhancement and depression in activity produced by combinations of stimuli is characteristic of superior colliculus neurons and is based on factors that generally signal the presence or absence of a meaningful relationship among those stimuli. For example, stimuli that occur at the same time and place are likely to be interrelated by common causality and to produce enhancement, while those that occur at different times and/or in different places are unlikely to be related and will produce depression (or no interaction). Although an individual's experience with specific cues is likely to alter their general effectiveness, so far there is no reason to suppose that it can change the interaction of a stimulus combination from enhancement to depression. Rather, experience plays its most essential role in aligning the different sensory maps in the superior colliculus (see chapter 12). Once the maps are aligned, neuronal enhancement or depression becomes dependent on the spatial and temporal relationships among stimuli. Stated another way, once the different sensory maps in the superior colliculus are aligned, multisensory interactions will depend on whether or not the stimuli are likely to have common causality. Such a system may have flaws, but it seems to work remarkably well.

RESPONSE ENHANCEMENT

Vigorous responses can be evoked from superior colliculus neurons with a single sensory cue, but their magnitude and reliability pale in comparison to responses evoked by combinations of sensory stimuli. In our experience, stimulus combinations produce significant increases over unimodal responses in every measure of activity one can evaluate using extracellular recording techniques: response reliability, number of impulses evoked, peak impulse frequency, and duration of the discharge train. An example of an enhanced response is shown in figure 10.1. This neuron was not special in any way we could determine on first inspection, and it responded, albeit poorly, to both moving and stationary visual stimuli. After repeated tests with light spots and bars of different sizes, moved at different velocities and in different direc-

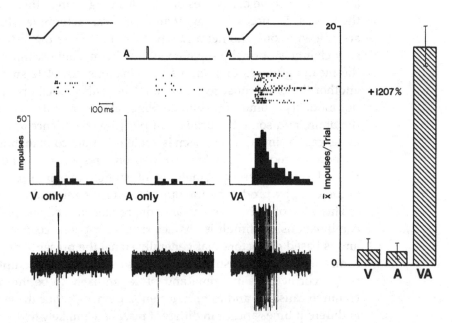

Figure 10.1 Visual-auditory response enhancement. A visual stimulus (V) evoked responses on only 6 of 16 trials in this neuron, and these responses were composed of few impulses. Responses are displayed in the rasters (1 dot = 1 impulse, each row = 1 trial), histograms, and representative oscillograms below the stimulus traces. An auditory stimulus (A) also evoked weak and unreliable responses. However, their combination produced a vigorous response on every trial. The mean number of impulses was increased by 1207% over that elicited by the most effective unimodal stimulus (vertical lines through bars = standard errors of the mean). These conventions are used in subsequent figures. (From Meredith and Stein 1986a)

tions, appropriate visual parameters were defined and the stimulus was presented 16 times in succession. The visual stimulus was not particularly effective, and responses were composed of few impulses and on many trials were absent altogether. Auditory stimuli were even less effective, and we could find no auditory stimulus that would activate the neuron on every trial. The best auditory stimulus was a brief hiss (100 msec duration sound), but it, too, was only marginally effective. However, when the weakly effective visual stimulus was combined with the nearly ineffective auditory stimulus, a very strong response was produced. The neuron's response was now far more reliable, and it was composed of a statistically significant increase in the number of impulses over that evoked by any visual or auditory stimulus alone.

Presumably, any such significant change in neuronal behavior resulting from combining sensory stimuli is detectable, that is, it stands out from background activity and can influence overt behavior. To assess the magnitude of each response enhancement produced by the combination of sensory stimuli, a simple formula is used that calculates the average number of impulses evoked by the most effective unimodal stimulus and compares it to the average number of impulses evoked by the combination of stimuli. As an example, let's say the most effective unimodal stimulus produced 4 impulses, but the multisensory stimulus produced 20 impulses. Therefore, according to our formula a 400% enhancement was produced by combining the two stimuli.

$$((CM - SM_{max}) \times 100)/SM_{max}$$

where CM = the number of impulses evoked by the combined-modality stimulus and SM_{max} = the response to the most effective single-modality stimulus.

Response enhancements are evident in every multisensory category (e.g., visual-auditory [figure 10.1], somatosensory-auditory [figure 10.2], somatosensory-visual [figure 10.3], and trimodal [figure 10.4]). However, it is not always immediately apparent that a neuron is multisensory. In some cases the influence of a sensory input becomes apparent only when it is combined with others: when presented alone it has no obvious effect on the neuron's activity, but it dramatically alters the neuron's responses to other inputs.

Most provocative are the examples in which activity is induced by combining two seemingly ineffective stimuli, as shown in figure 10.4. In these examples neither stimulus alone is capable of evoking superior colliculus–mediated behavior, because neither is capable of producing propagated action potentials in superior colliculus neurons; yet as a combined stimulus they can and do produce action potentials. This dramatically illustrates the potent effect of combinations of sensory stimuli, an effect that undoubtedly is a common occurrence in more typical environmental contexts.

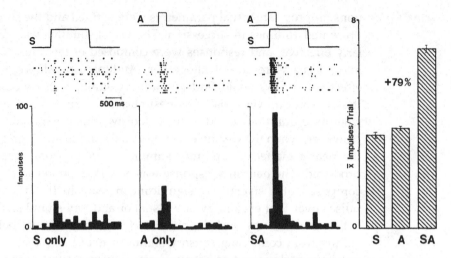

Figure 10.2 Somatosensory-auditory response enhancement. A unimodal somatosensory or auditory stimulus produced few responses, but their combination significantly enhanced this neuron's responsiveness. (From Meredith and Stein 1986a)

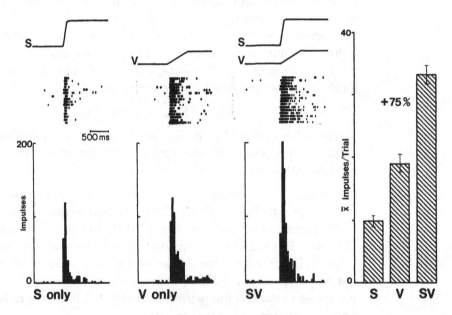

Figure 10.3 Somatosensory-visual response enhancement. (From Meredith and Stein 1986a)

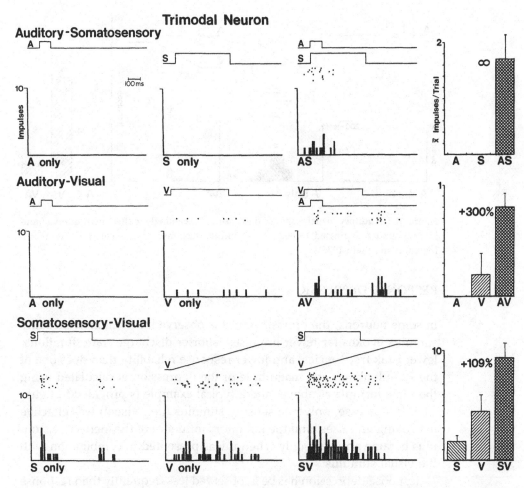

Figure 10.4 Combining any two unimodal stimuli can enhance responses in trimodal neurons. Although auditory and somatosensory stimuli presented alone were insufficient to activate this neuron (*top row*), combining these stimuli evoked responses in 8 of 10 trials. Similarly, an auditory stimulus that was ineffective alone enhanced the weak responses to the visual stimulus (*center row*). Other unimodal somatosensory and visual stimuli proved to be more effective (*bottom row*), but their combination still increased response reliability and magnitude. (From Meredith and Stein 1986a)

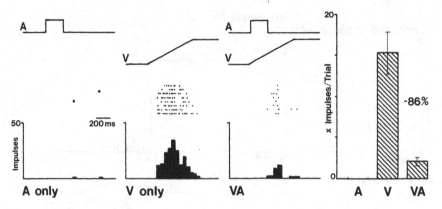

Figure 10.5 Auditory-visual response depression. A seemingly ineffective auditory stimulus profoundly depressed (−86%) this neuron's response to a visual stimulus. (From Meredith and Stein 1986a)

RESPONSE DEPRESSION

In some neurons, the opposite effect is observed: a combined-modality stimulus evokes far fewer impulses, shorter discharge train durations, lower peak frequencies, and lower response reliability than does one of the stimuli alone. The magnitude of the depression is calculated using the same formula as above, and a typical example is provided in figure 10.5. In this case, only one sensory stimulus (i.e., visual) was effective in evoking impulses, and the inhibitory influence of the ineffective stimulus became apparent only when it was presented in combination with the visual stimulus.

Response depression has been observed less frequently than response enhancement and seems to be dependent on the presence of such specific receptive field properties as spatial inhibition, inhibitory surrounds, or inhibitory monaural inputs (see chapter 5 for a review of receptive field properties). Apparently, while every multisensory receptive field has an excitatory region, and therefore holds the potential for enhancement, not all have the spatial characteristic (i.e., an inhibitory surround) necessary to produce multisensory inhibition.

SPACE AND TIME: RULES GOVERNING MULTISENSORY INTEGRATION ARE BASED ON UNIMODAL RECEPTIVE FIELD CHARACTERISTICS

Rather than being immutable characteristics of a particular neuron, multisensory enhancement and depression proved to be determined by the spatial and temporal characteristics of the stimuli. By manipulating these parameters, the same combinations of stimuli can produce response enhancement or depression in the same neuron. In fact, very simple rules govern the nature and magnitude of multisensory integration, and these rules are based on a neuron's unimodal receptive field characteristics.

Space

Spatially coincident multisensory stimuli tend to produce response enhancement, whereas spatially disparate stimuli produce either depression or no interaction.

During the initial observations of multisensory enhancement in superior colliculus neurons it was thought possible that the great increase in responses to stimulus combinations reflected a generalized arousal phenomenon. The very presence of multiple stimuli might have aroused greater activity throughout the brain by increasing neuronal sensitivity to any and all stimuli. By varying the positions of the different sensory stimuli and evaluating their effects on multisensory integration, it soon became apparent that this was not the case. Enhancement was not due to a generalized effect on the brain, or to a generalized effect on these neurons, but was evident only when the stimuli followed a rather clear-cut spatial rule: it occurred only when combinations of sensory stimuli were presented within their respective receptive fields. A visual-auditory stimulus pair had to have the visual stimulus within the visual receptive field and the auditory stimulus within the auditory receptive field. Because the different receptive fields of a multisensory neuron overlap, stimuli located near one another in space enhance one another's effects. Although this is most evident in visual-auditory neurons because both representations in the superior colliculus refer to "out there" in extrapersonal space, the same is also true for the visual-somatosensory and auditory-somatosensory representations. The representational axes of all three modalities are the same (this can be seen by using the composite map of sensory space shown in figure 8.2), so that, for example, visual and auditory stimuli directly in front of the animal's face will occur in spatial register with tactile stimuli on the face, and vice versa. These conditions of multisensory spatial register lead to response enhancements.

On the other hand, when one sensory stimulus was positioned so that it was outside the borders of its receptive field, it not only failed to enhance the effect of a second stimulus within its receptive field, but, in many neurons, it actually depressed responses to the excitatory stimulus. Often the depression was quite dramatic, eliminating even vigorous responses that had been elicited by every presentation of the first (i.e., excitatory) stimulus.

The spatial property of multisensory integration is readily understandable in terms of the organization of zones of excitation and inhibition that define a receptive field. Operationally, receptive fields are defined by an enclosed region in which a sensory stimulus produces excitation. Sometimes, however, these excitatory zones are bordered by inhibitory areas that act to antagonize the effect of a stimulus within the excitatory zone. An example of this is shown in figure 10.6. Activation of the inhibitory surround produces a generalized inhibition, regardless of the stimulus modality. It suppresses all excitatory inputs to that neuron, even those originating from other sensory modalities. Yet, there is nothing intrinsically inhibitory about the stimulus itself (or excitatory about the other), and it will exist simultaneously within the receptive fields of other neurons and have an excitatory influence on those neurons. Similarly, the excitatory stimulus in this example will exist simultaneously in the inhibitory zones of other neurons and have an inhibitory influence on their activity. The overt behavior that results from these combinations of stimuli depends on the product of multisensory interactions in the entire population of neurons. In the simplest scheme, the inhibition generated by the stronger of two disparate stimuli will render the weaker stimulus ineffective, while retaining much of its own excitatory influence. The result is likely to be the animal's selective attention and orientation to the stronger of the two stimuli.

The example provided in figure 10.7 illustrates the enhanced and depressed interaction discussed above, but also reveals that enhancement can be produced even when the visual and the auditory stimuli are not in exactly the same position in space. Because the requirement for enhancement is simply that the stimuli be within their respective receptive fields, the presence of large receptive fields, especially in multisensory neurons, provides a good deal of latitude in the exact positions the two stimuli must occupy in space in order to enhance one another. Since there is rarely an exact spatial correspondence of receptive fields for any individual neuron, it may well be that in some cases optimal enhancement would even require a slight separation among stimuli.

The fact that the receptive field, and not space, is the proper referent for multisensory integration is particularly evident in the rather strange receptive fields in which multiple excitatory regions are separated by ineffective zones. One example is the visual-somatosensory neuron shown in figure 10.8. Its somatosensory excitatory regions include the forepaw and hindpaw, but not the intervening body. Visual responses are enhanced when a tactile stimulus is presented on either the forepaw or hindpaw, but not when it is presented on the intervening body. Since enhancement depends on stimuli being within an excitatory receptive field, one would correctly predict that if a "receptive field" encompasses all of sensory space, a stimulus anywhere in this space would produce enhancement. The applicability of the spatial rule to somatosensory-auditory neurons is shown in figure 10.9.

These examples are presented to make a significant point: the fact that stimuli from the same region in space produce response enhancement appears to be a consequence of the alignment of sensory maps. Of

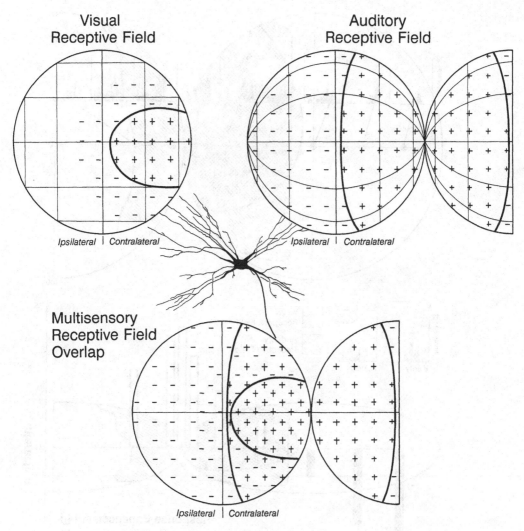

Visual
Receptive Field

Ipsilateral | *Contralateral*

Auditory
Receptive Field

Ipsilateral | *Contralateral*

Multisensory
Receptive Field
Overlap

Ipsilateral | *Contralateral*

Figure 10.6 Excitatory and inhibitory regions of a prototypical multisensory neuron. Excitatory visual (*top left*) and auditory (*top right*) receptive fields are often surrounded by inhibitory regions. When these receptive fields are superimposed (*bottom*), it is evident that a spatially coincident multisensory stimulus can evoke pure excitation from only a restricted region of space (dense pluses), while antagonism (plus-minus) or inhibition (minuses) would occur when stimuli occurred elsewhere.

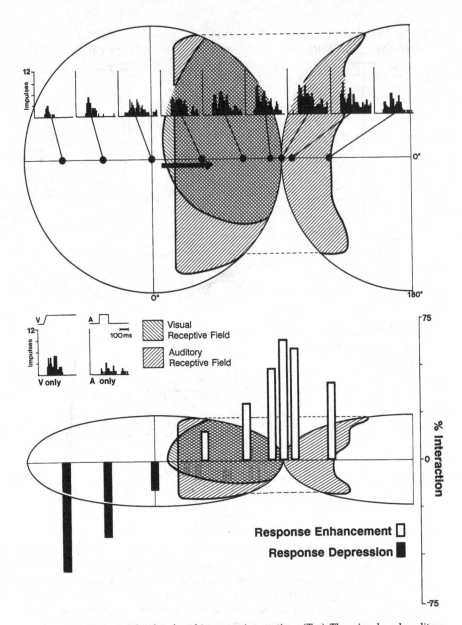

Figure 10.7 The spatial rule of multisensory integration. (*Top*) The visual and auditory receptive fields of this bimodal neuron overlap one another. A visual stimulus (arrow) was presented in combination with an auditory stimulus at each location marked by a filled circle. Their multisensory responses are presented in histograms above (representative unimodal responses are shown below the receptive field drawings). These data are summarized in the perspective drawing at the bottom, where a third axis has been added: the magnitude of the response interaction. Note that the auditory stimulus significantly enhanced responses to the visual stimulus whenever it was within its receptive field, but significantly depressed response to the visual stimulus when it fell outside its receptive field (also see figure 10.6).

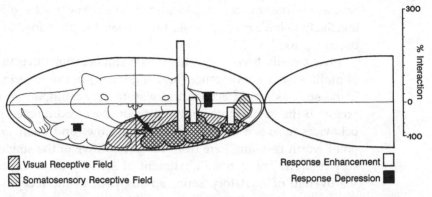

Visual Receptive Field
Somatosensory Receptive Field

Response Enhancement
Response Depression

Figure 10.8 The spatial rule applies to visual-somatosensory neurons. Response enhancement was evoked in this bimodal neuron only when the visual and somatosensory stimuli were within their receptive fields. When the somatosensory stimulus was outside its receptive field it was unable to significantly alter responses to the visual stimulus.

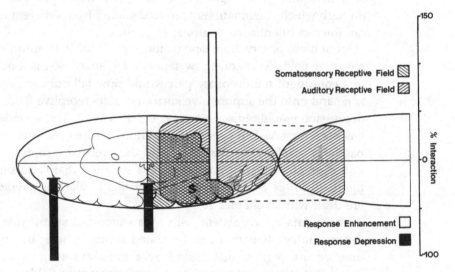

Somatosensory Receptive Field
Auditory Receptive Field

Response Enhancement
Response Depression

Figure 10.9 The spatial rule applies to somatosensory-auditory neurons. Response enhancement was evoked in this bimodal neuron only when the somatosensory and auditory stimuli were within their receptive fields. When the auditory stimulus was moved outside its receptive field, to the midline or ipsilateral auditory space, it depressed responses to the somatosensory stimulus.

course, for intersensory map alignment to have evolved in the first place it is likely to have made it easier for animals to obtain food and to avoid becoming food.

It has already been suggested on several occasions that the presence of multisensory convergence (and alignment) in the superior colliculus is the simplest, most economical way to give multiple sensory inputs access to the same motor outputs to produce coordinated orientation behaviors (also see Stein et al. 1976b; Gaither and Stein 1979). It is a point worth restating here from the perspective of the single multisensory neuron. The general alignment of sensory maps is produced by the overlap of excitatory zones among each of the receptive fields of the multisensory neurons that constitute them, a consequence that is unlikely to be serendipitous. In the world beyond the laboratory, multisensory stimuli that are derived from the same event are also derived from the same point in space, as in the example of the sight and sound of a mosquito. The alignment of receptive fields provides a means through which combinations of related stimuli from different modalities can interact to enhance neuronal responses.

From these observations one would expect that if a neuron's different receptive fields were somehow separated in space, so that one stimulus of a coincident multisensory pair would now fall outside its excitatory zone and onto the suppressive surround of its receptive field, response depression would replace response enhancement. This is, indeed, what has been observed in experimental animals when the ears or eyes are passively displaced so that they, and their related receptive fields, are no longer aligned with one another, a situation that is documented in figure 10.10 (possible consequences of this in alert, behaving animals are dealt with in chapter 13).

These data are consistent with a parsimonious spatial rule of multisensory integration that can be stated formally here: Because of the intersensory register maintained by a multisensory neuron, spatially coincident stimuli fall within its excitatory receptive fields and enhance one another's effects. However, if the stimuli are disparate, one may fall within the inhibitory receptive region and depress the effects of the other.

Time

Maximal multisensory interactions are not dependent on matching the onset of two different sensory stimuli, or their latencies, but on how the activity patterns resulting from the two inputs overlap.

Some of the temporal restrictions on multisensory integration are quite obvious: stimuli occurring in close temporal proximity affect one another, while those separated by long intervals are processed as separate events. Two unexpected results of the studies examining these temporal

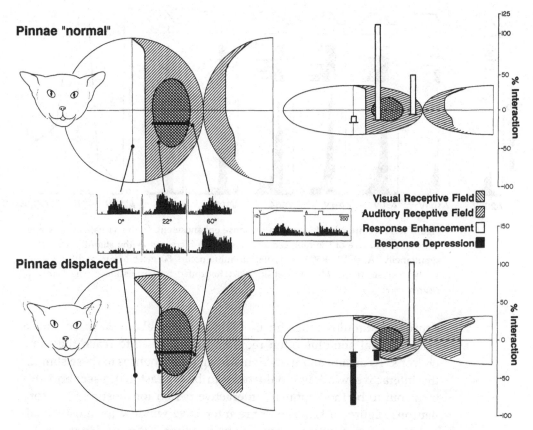

Pinnae "normal"

0° 22° 60°

Pinnae displaced

Visual Receptive Field
Auditory Receptive Field
Response Enhancement
Response Depression

% Interaction

Figure 10.10 Effect of misaligning sensory organs on multisensory integration. In the example shown here, the most effective visual (arrow)-auditory (filled circles) combination was obtained with the auditory stimulus at 22° from midline (see middle histogram and perspective drawing at right). However, when the ears were deviated to the contralateral side ("pinnae displaced") the auditory receptive field shifted approximately 30° contralaterally, and so did the position of the most effective visual-auditory combination (60°). The former best position now fell outside the auditory receptive field, and an auditory stimulus there depressed responses to the visual (see perspective drawing, lower right).

restrictions were the long duration of the "temporal window" within which interactions can occur and the observation that stimuli matched for their physical onset or their latencies to activate the same neurons do not necessarily produce the most intense interactions.

Upon reflection, the wide temporal window makes excellent sense. Since the modalities must deal with environmental energies that travel at radically different velocities (e.g., light = 186,000 mi/sec; sound = 1100 ft/sec or 0.21 mi/sec), the inputs from the same event reach the peripheral sensory organs at very different times. Even after they reach the proper receptors there are substantial differences in the processing and conduction times to the central nervous system and thus to the individual multisensory neurons. An auditory stimulus presented close to the ear takes approximately 13 msec to activate a superior colliculus

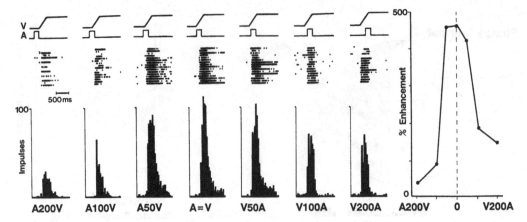

Figure 10.11 Temporal influences on response enhancement. In this visual-auditory neuron, the magnitude of the multisensory interaction increased as the stimuli approached simultaneity (A = V). V50A = visual stimulus occurs 50 msec before auditory; A50V = the reverse. (From Meredith et al. 1987. Reprinted by permission of the *Journal of Neuroscience*)

neuron, a stimulus touching the skin averages about 26 msec, and a nearby visual stimulus often requires 65–100 msec to reach the same neurons. To ensure an interaction among the responses to these stimuli, the interactive window would have to be at least 100 msec, and this turns out to be the "optimal" interactive period for most multisensory neurons (figure 10.11). The entire interactive window for most visual-somatosensory neurons appears to be less than 250 msec. However, for visual-auditory neurons, because both the auditory and visual systems are specialized for the detection of distant events, which reach the superior colliculus far earlier through the eye than the ear, a far broader interactive window is sometimes necessary if visual-auditory interactions are to take place. We have found some visual-auditory neurons in which interactions can take place for periods of up to 1500 msec, which, given the rather short time periods over which neural responses to transient visual, auditory, and innocuous somatosensory stimuli are believed to exist, is an extraordinarily long time.

The determinant of the interactive period is the duration of the effect a stimulus induces, and this includes its effects on the neuron's membrane characteristics. If, for example, a visual stimulus evokes a train of discharges lasting 200 msec, auditory inputs arriving anywhere within that 200-msec period will interact with the visually induced activity. If there is an additional period after the visual discharge during which the cell's membrane characteristics are affected, the interactive period will be even longer. In such a case the effects of a late-arriving auditory input may still be altered by the changed membrane properties induced by the earlier visual stimulus.

Because each input produces a train of activity that varies over time, the effect of one input on another will differ depending on their temporal relationship. This might, of course, also vary depending on the properties of different neurons. In the population of neurons examined thus far, some enhancements were found to be maximal when the two inputs arrived simultaneously; however, quite often this was not the case. Instead, the key for enhancement was the overlap of the peak discharge periods of the two stimuli, as shown in figure 10.12, and often this did not occur when the two stimuli were presented simultaneously.

Inhibitory periods usually cannot be monitored using extracellular electrodes; the stimulus simply appears to be ineffective and the neuron does not discharge. Nevertheless, the logic of maximizing depression is the same as that for maximizing enhancement. By trial and success one can adjust the onset of an inhibitory stimulus to achieve maximal effectiveness. Presumably, this is the result of overlapping the peak inhibitory period with the peak excitatory period produced by the other stimulus. Generally, peak levels of depression, like those of enhancement, are elicited when an inhibitory stimulus is presented within 100 msec of an excitatory stimulus (figure 10.13).

Curiously, in some neurons, varying the interval between stimuli can reverse the sign of an interaction and convert enhancement to depression (figure 10.14). Examination of the unimodal discharge trains evoked by one or both of the stimuli has revealed the presence of postexcitatory inhibitory periods. In neurons with reasonably high spontaneous firing rates, this is apparent as a reduction in activity. When the postexcitatory inhibitory period evoked by one stimulus overlaps the excitatory period of the other stimulus, it reduces its effectiveness—a form of proactive inhibition induced by a stimulus that on first examination seems only excitatory. However, response depression that is induced by spatially disparate stimuli cannot be converted into response enhancement by changing the temporal interval between stimuli (figure 10.15).

These observations illustrate the complex nature of the integration of inputs from multiple sensory stimuli that take place over time. Yet, the two temporal features that characterize the multisensory interactions in superior colliculus neurons can be stated quite simply: (1) the interactive windows can be very long, and (2) overlapping the peak activity (excitatory or inhibitory) periods produced by two unimodal stimuli maximizes their interactions.

The presence of these features hardly seems coincidental. Quite the contrary, they are likely to have developed and been maintained during evolution because: (1) the presence of wide temporal windows gives critical flexibility in detecting and responding to minimal, albeit important stimuli at different distances from the animal (figure 10.16), and (2) the appearance of maximal depression when spatially disparate stimuli are in close temporal proximity is a means of focusing attention on the strongest, and presumably the most important, stimulus in the presence of potential distractors. Both effects have an impact on vertebrate

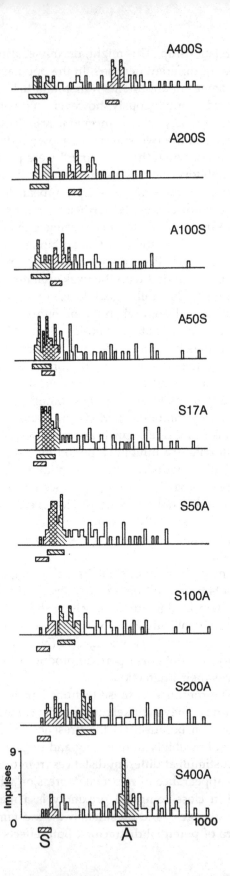

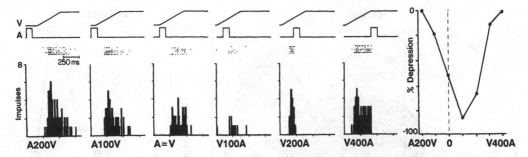

Figure 10.13 Temporal influences on response depression. When the visual stimulus was initiated 100 msec before an ipsilateral auditory stimulus, its effectiveness was maximally depressed. The ability of the auditory stimulus to depress visual responses decayed as the temporal disparity between the stimuli was increased or decreased from this optimum (see graph). (From Meredith et al. 1987. Reprinted by permission of the *Journal of Neuroscience*)

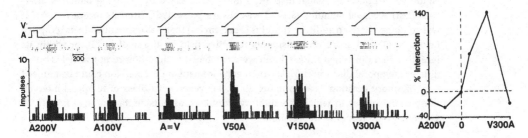

Figure 10.14 Changing the temporal interval between stimuli can change enhancement to depression. Unimodal auditory and visual stimuli were each effective in activating this neuron, and combining these stimuli at some intervals (V50A, V150A) produced response enhancement. However, at longer intervals (A200V, V300A) the combination produced the opposite effect: fewer impulses than a single-modality stimulus (i.e., response depression). These effects are summarized in the graph (right). (From Meredith et al. 1987. Reprinted by permission of the *Journal of Neuroscience*)

◀ Figure 10.12 Peak enhancement is achieved by overlapping peak unimodal discharge periods. In this auditory-somatosensory neuron, stimulus combinations presented at 400, 200, and 100 msec intervals were processed as separate events. Shorter interstimulus intervals (A50S, S50A) evoked discharge trains whose peak periods of activity (hatched areas) overlapped (cross-hatched areas) and generated significant levels of response enhancement (+167% and +131%, respectively). Near-simultaneous (S17A) stimulus presentation produced the maximal overlap of peak activity periods and, thereby, produced maximal levels of enhancement (+181%). (From Meredith et al. 1987. Reprinted by permission of the *Journal of Neuroscience*)

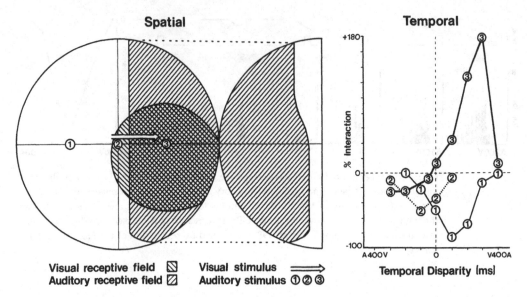

Spatial　　　　　　　　　　　**Temporal**

Visual receptive field ⊠　　Visual stimulus ⟹
Auditory receptive field ⊟　Auditory stimulus ① ② ③

Temporal Disparity (ms)

Figure 10.15 Effects of spatial disparity cannot be reversed by changing temporal intervals. (*Left*) A visual stimulus (arrow) was always presented within its receptive field. It was combined with an auditory stimulus (open circles) that was either outside its receptive field in ipsilateral space (1), outside its receptive field on the midline (2), or within its receptive field (3). When these stimuli were combined within their receptive fields but at different temporal disparities (*right*), both enhancement and depression could be induced (e.g., auditory position 3) as in figure 10.14. However, regardless of temporal interval, those combinations in which the auditory stimulus was outside its receptive field (1, 2) generated only response depression.

viability, and are likely to have been major factors in their survival and proliferation. It is not inconceivable that similar features play a significant role in the survival of invertebrate species as well.

RECEPTIVE FIELD PROPERTIES AND MULTISENSORY INTEGRATION

Receptive field properties are neither created nor eliminated by combining inputs from different sensory systems.

Receptive field properties act as neuronal filters, determining which stimuli will activate a neuron and how vigorous that activation will be. In effect, they provide a means of selecting which stimuli gain access to which circuits, and in this case determine the stimuli that can effect attentive and orientation responses via the superior colliculus. It would complicate matters enormously if there were significant changes in receptive field properties with every change in circumstance. Fortunately, within very broad limits this does not seem to occur, at least not with the changes in responsiveness that are induced by combining different sensory stimuli.

An example of the robustness of unimodal receptive field characteris-

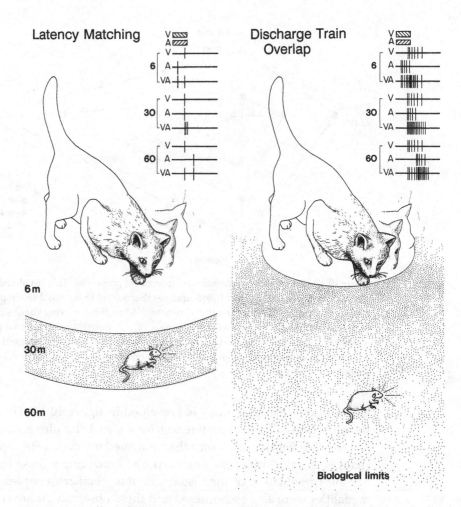

Latency Matching

V 〰️
A ▨

6	V
	A
	VA

30	V
	A
	VA

60	V
	A
	VA

Discharge Train Overlap

V 〰️
A ▨

6	V
	A
	VA

30	V
	A
	VA

60	V
	A
	VA

6 m

30 m

60 m

6 m

Biological limits

Figure 10.16 Effect of basing multisensory interactions on overlapping discharge trains, rather than matching latencies. There are significant differences among the modalities in the speed with which inputs reach the receptors and the conduction time from receptors to central neurons. If interactions could occur only when input latencies are matched, integration in visual-auditory neurons would occur only when the cues originate from a narrow strip 7–39 meters from the cat (shaded area). Note that in this case (see the schematized oscillograms above the cat's head), when the stimuli are at 30 meters their inputs produce more than the simple addition of impulses that occurs at 6 and 60 meters. However, interactions can occur as long as any portion of the two unimodal discharge trains (or their periods of altered membrane potential) overlap. This extends the interactive window, and integration of auditory-visual stimuli can take place at varying distances from the observer. (From Meredith et al. 1987. Reprinted by permission of the *Journal of Neuroscience*)

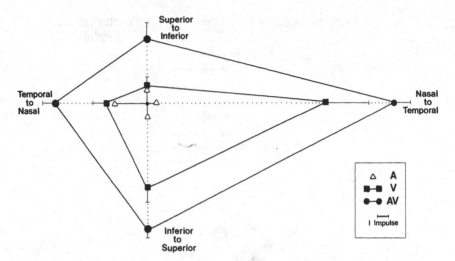

Figure 10.17 Preservation of unimodal receptive field properties. This visual-auditory neuron preferred a visual stimulus (filled squares) that moved in the nasal-to-temporal direction above those that moved in other directions. When these moving visual stimuli were combined with a stationary auditory stimulus (filled circles), this directional preference remained despite a striking change in responsiveness. Open triangles represent responses to the stationary auditory stimulus that were interleaved during trials in which the visual stimulus was moved.

tics in multisensory neurons is presented in figure 10.17. This neuron showed strong direction preferences for a visual stimulus moved across its receptive field, a preference that remained intact despite several-fold changes in responsiveness produced by introducing a noise burst during the presentation of the visual stimulus. Similar examples in other modalities were also encountered and these observations are consistent with the results of the spatial and temporal experiments described earlier: the borders of unimodal receptive fields and their discharge trains determine the multisensory product.

Apparently, then, integration of multiple cues increases or decreases the signal in the superior colliculus (and presumably the likelihood of an overt response), but does not alter the fundamentals of the filters. Consequently, a stimulus such as color, which is not normally effective in activating superior colliculus neurons, will not suddenly become a potent stimulus when coupled, for example, with an auditory stimulus, nor will superior colliculus neurons become better discriminators of pitch because tactile and auditory stimuli are paired.

UNIMODAL AND MULTISENSORY INTEGRATION ARE NOT EQUIVALENT

The multiplicative interactions that characterize superior colliculus responses to two stimuli from different modalities are not apparent when the stimuli are from the same modality.

Despite the fact that multisensory integration depends on unimodal responses and unimodal receptive field properties, one cannot assume that the consequences of pairing two stimuli from the same modality (e.g., two spots of light next to each other) will match those of pairing stimuli from different modalities. In the instances we have investigated, these different combinations appear to produce quite different results.

Pairs of unimodal stimuli never result in the same sort of multiplicative response enhancement that combinations of multisensory stimuli do. Although the combination of two excitatory stimuli from the same modality generally does produce an increase in the firing rate of the neuron, it is less than the number of impulses that would occur if their individual products are simply added together: a response "occlusion." In some cases it actually decreases the firing rate of the neuron from that evoked by one stimulus, an inhibitory effect previously noted by researchers examining the effects of pairing within-modality stimuli on cortical evoked potentials (see chapter 1) and in single neuron studies in monkey temporal cortex (see Sato 1989). In contrast, when stimuli from different modalities are combined, even in the same neurons in which unimodal pairs produce inhibition, a multisensory enhancement results in which the product usually far exceeds the sum of the impulses evoked by the individual stimuli. An example is provided in figure 10.18.

MULTISENSORY INTERACTIONS AND STIMULUS EFFECTIVENESS

Maximal enhancement occurs with minimally effective stimuli.

The magnitude of response enhancement varies widely among neurons and even within the same neuron when different stimulus parameters are used. But in general, a very simple inverse relationship exists between the effectiveness of the stimuli and the responses evoked: combinations of weak unimodal stimuli produce the greatest enhancements.

An example of this phenomenon is demonstrated for one neuron in figure 10.19. For this neuron, as for most others examined, the unimodal stimuli that evoked the greatest number of impulses when presented alone also evoked the greatest number of impulses when combined. However, the percentage change in activity produced by that stimulus combination was also the lowest. The opposite was true for the least effective unimodal stimuli; they produced the lowest number of impulses when presented alone, but the highest percentage enhancement in combination. The enhancement relationship is, of course, always a comparative one, and it has become evident that the combination of stimuli produces some multiple of the activity evoked by the most effective unimodal stimulus when presented alone. In its most dramatic form this relationship allows two stimuli that are ineffective individually to become effective when combined (see figure 10.4). Sometimes the resul-

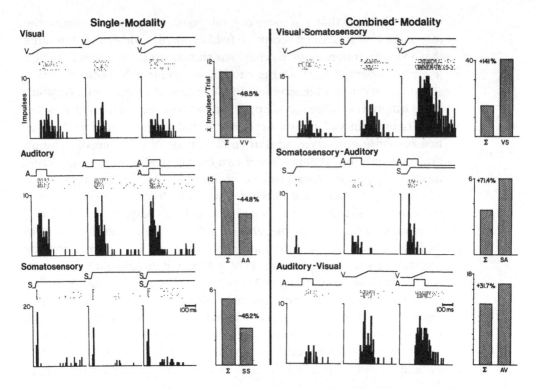

Figure 10.18 Unimodal and multisensory integration differ. When unimodal pairs of stimuli were combined (*left*: visual-visual, auditory-auditory, somatosensory-somatosensory), the responses evoked were consistently less than the sum of those produced by the individual stimuli. However, when stimuli from different modalities were paired (*right*), the responses were consistently greater than that sum.

tant activity in such cases is surprisingly vigorous. Since the absolute magnitude of the comparative change, and even its sign (from positive to negative), can be varied systematically by manipulating the parameters of the unimodal stimuli, familiar descriptive terms such as "occlusion," "summation," and "facilitation" have been avoided here. While these terms themselves are not incorrect, they give the erroneous impression that static categories can be used in classifying dynamic effects that fall along continua.

But regardless of how one describes the multiplicative changes in activity that occur by combining stimuli, the next question raised is, How does it occur at the neuronal level? Unfortunately, at this point we really do not know, but one possibility is that some ion channels in the neuronal membrane remain closed in the presence of unimodal inputs but are opened by the combination of multiple sensory inputs, thereby producing an amplified response in the neuron. The most obvious candidate for mediating such an effect is a receptor coupled to a voltage-sensitive channel. Current fascination with the *N*-methyl-D-aspartate (NMDA) receptor brings it to mind immediately. It would be of great interest to determine if NMDA agonists (and antagonists) can

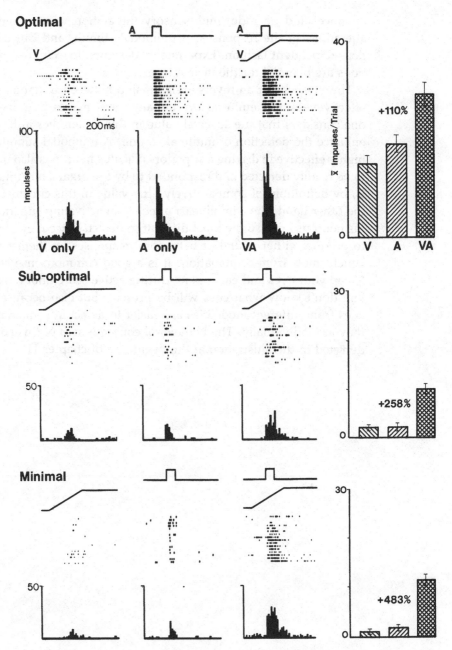

Figure 10.19 Multisensory enhancement increases as unimodal stimulus effectiveness decreases. As the physical parameters of the single-modality stimuli are systematically changed (e.g., size of the visual [V] stimulus, intensity of the auditory stimulus [A]), so that progressively fewer discharges are evoked, the percentage of response enhancement resulting from their combination increases. (From Meredith and Stein 1986a)

enhance (and degrade) multisensory integration with minimal or no alterations in the responses to unimodal stimuli, and can do so in a dose-dependent fashion. Experiments designed to examine these questions are planned for the near future.

The presence of an inverse relationship between unimodal stimulus effectiveness and multisensory enhancement makes intuitive sense if one considers that the survival value in this system lies in its ability to enhance the detection of minimal stimuli. A unimodal stimulus that is highly effective in driving a superior colliculus neuron is also most likely to be readily detected and responded to by the organism. Amplification is, by definition, of comparatively little value in this circumstance. On the other hand, the stimuli least effective in activating superior colliculus neurons are also the most difficult to detect. Since they are unlikely to produce either neural or behavioral responses by themselves, they benefit most from combination. It is a good commonsense strategy to "keep your eyes and ears open" during active search not only because you don't know what cues will be present, but also because minimal cues from different modalities are easier to detect in combination than they are individually. The behavioral consequences of this concept are depicted in the illustration at the beginning of chapter 11.

11 Behavioral Consequences of Multisensory Interactions

Electrophysiological Experiments with Awake Animals

What has been discussed thus far is how multisensory integration affects the sensory responses of superior colliculus neurons. Presumably this sensory integration has a potent effect on the premotor discharges of superior colliculus neurons that are closely linked to the initiation of a movement. While premotor neurons have been studied intensively in behaving animals, surprisingly little has been learned about the consequences of multisensory stimuli on premotor activity. Nevertheless, it is evident that visual as well as nonvisual stimuli have access to visuomotor premotor neurons, not only because most multisensory neurons are descending efferents (Meredith and Stein 1985, 1986a), but because neurons unequivocally demonstrated to be visuomotor in behaving animals can be affected by nonvisual stimuli (Jay and Sparks 1987b; Peck 1987). For example, visual as well as auditory stimuli were shown to activate visuomotor neurons in the superior colliculus, thereby allowing the eyes to acquire visual and auditory targets. Presumably, the same is true of somatosensory stimuli.

Multisensory enhancement and depression change the firing frequency and the durations of the discharge trains of sensory responses, thereby increasing or decreasing the salience of the event. In premotor neurons, however, firing frequency and discharge duration are not directly linked to stimulus salience, but are coupled to the metrics of a movement. In visuomotor neurons they code the velocity and distance the eye will move (Mays and Sparks 1980; Munoz and Guitton 1985; Berthoz et al. 1986). Undoubtedly, then, the motor discharges initiated by multisensory inputs are not a faithful reproduction of the sensory responses, but represent a transformation of them into a motor coordinate system. Thus far only one report (Peck 1987) has examined the integrative effect of multisensory stimuli on neurons identified as premotor. A neuron in the cat superior colliculus that initially failed to meet the criteria of a *pre*motor neuron in response to unimodal stimuli (it fired only *after* the onset of an eye movement initiated by a visual or an auditory stimulus) did meet the criteria when the animal was presented with the combination of these stimuli. Now the neuron was recruited to discharge *before* an eye movement, and, presumably, to aid in its initiation. If enough neurons respond in this fashion, the probability of overt behavior will increase.

Obviously, far more information is needed before we can understand how integrated multisensory signals are transformed into the motor commands that coordinate the overt responses mediated by the superior colliculus. However, a good deal of information is now available about the elicitation of overt attentive and orientation responses by multisensory stimuli in paradigms very much like those used to study the neural events described earlier.

BEHAVIORAL EXPERIMENTS WITH TRAINED ANIMALS

Figure 11.1 was originally drawn to represent what is believed to be one of the primary adaptive advantages of multisensory enhancement in the superior colliculus: facilitating attentive and orientation responses to minimally effective stimuli that occur together in space. This figure illustrates the most straightforward behavioral predictions that can be made

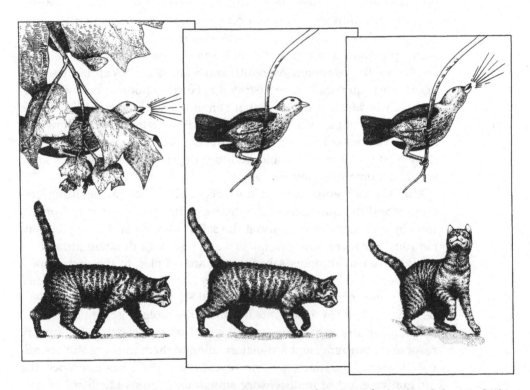

Figure 11.1 Multisensory stimuli can enhance detection and orientation behaviors. In this hypothetical situation, a bird whose song or image is within the cat's auditory (*left*) or visual (*center*) field fails to evoke an orientation response. However, when the two cues are combined (*right*), the neural activity elicited is sufficient to exceed the threshold for an overt response.

on the basis of the electrophysiological data. But, are they correct? At the time they were set forth it was impossible to say, because despite the realization of one of our original aims—describing some of the neural bases of multisensory integration—the behavioral correlates of these particular predictions had not been demonstrated. Therefore, it was necessary to examine whether the rules governing multisensory integration at the level of the single superior colliculus neuron are applicable to the overt responses of an intact, behaving animal.

A simple paradigm, designed to be similar to that used to study the behavior of single neurons, was used to examine how cats would attend and orient to unimodal and multisensory stimuli (Stein et al. 1988, 1989). Each animal was required to fixate directly ahead at what was labeled 0 degrees, and to walk directly to a stimulus which would occur at any of a variety of eccentricities, as shown in figure 11.2. Any response other than a brisk and direct approach to the correct stimulus was considered incorrect. The first objective was to establish how readily an animal would detect, orient to, and approach a unimodal stimulus (e.g., visual). The next step was to compare that behavior to the animal's ability to respond to that stimulus when it was paired with one from another modality (e.g., auditory) presented either at the same location or at successively greater spatial disparities.

It was expected that training animals to perform this task would be extremely easy. Unfortunately, there are significant differences between behavioral tests that are conceptually simple and tasks that cats will deign to perform. But after long training periods, the animals would

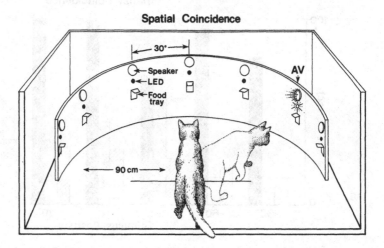

Figure 11.2 Behavioral paradigm for studying the consequences of spatially coincident multisensory stimuli. A speaker (large circle) and a light-emitting diode (LED, small circle) are located in vertical pairs above a food tray at each of seven regularly spaced (30°) intervals. During training and testing, an animal was required to orient to and move directly toward a visual and/or an auditory stimulus (e.g., 60° right) to receive a food reward. When the auditory and visual stimuli were presented simultaneously, they were at the same eccentricity. (From Stein et al. 1989)

stand quietly at the ready position fixating at 0 degrees, and reliably (95–100% of the trials) approach a comparatively intense unimodal stimulus at any of the positions tested. When they did so, they were rewarded with food. They were then ready to be tested with stimuli that were far more difficult to discern. The testing situation was divided into three paradigms, (1) spatially coincident trials, (2) spatially disparate trials, and (3) spatial resolution trials.

Spatially-Coincident Trials

In this paradigm, each animal was taught to approach a visual or an auditory stimulus regardless of its position. During testing, various stimulus intensities and positions were presented randomly. However, when the visual and the auditory stimuli were presented simultaneously, they were always at the same spatial location. As one would expect, the animals did poorest with unimodal stimuli of the lowest intensities presented at the most peripheral positions (they were also extremely difficult for human observers to detect). Incorrect responses generally consisted of a failure to move when the stimulus came on, as if the animal was unaware of its presence, or a wandering in the apparatus as if the animal was aware that something happened, but not where it happened.

The example presented in figure 11.3 is from a single animal and demonstrates the general phenomenon observed: comparatively few

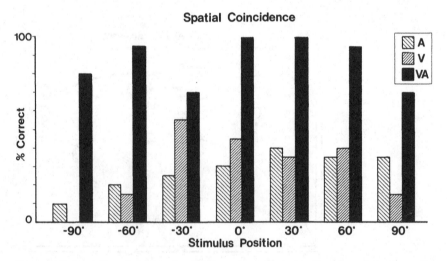

Figure 11.3 Spatially coincident stimuli enhance correct responding. Low-intensity auditory (A) and visual (V) stimuli were presented individually and then simultaneously (AV) at each of the seven eccentricities described in figure 11.2. The animal's ability to detect and approach the correct position was enhanced by combined-modality stimuli at every location. Stimulus position is shown in degrees (right = positive, left = negative). The same conventions are used in subsequent figures. (From Stein et al. 1989)

Multisensory Convergence and Integration at the Level of the Single Neuron low intensity single-modality stimuli were responded to correctly, but combining the two stimuli produced a multiplicative enhancement in correct responses. At −90 (90 degrees to the left of fixation) the visual stimulus never evoked a correct response and the auditory stimulus was responded to on only 10% of the trials. However, combining the two stimuli at this location enhanced correct responding well beyond that which would be predicted by statistical methods (see figure 11.6 for the formula used) or by the sum of responses to the individual cues. Similar enhancements, although of somewhat lower magnitude, were seen at all other eccentricities.

With only rare exceptions, the enhancement of correct responses with combined stimuli was observed in every animal and at every eccentricity and intensity at which single-modality stimuli evoked substantially less than perfect performance. However, the magnitude of the enhancement was greatest at the lowest intensities, where the probability of correctly responding to unimodal stimuli was lowest. At higher stimulus intensities, not only did the unimodal cues become consistently more effective, so that there was a decrease in the possible magnitude of enhancement, but the maximum possible enhancement was often not realized either. Thus, when the visual cue was sufficiently intense to produce 70–80% correct responses alone, the addition of the auditory cue often produced no further increment, thereby giving the impression that multisensory enhancement will not be evident with cues that are already highly effective. In contrast, the multiplicative nature of interactions with low-intensity stimuli reached their extreme in several cases in which the unimodal stimuli were rarely or never responded to correctly, but their combination was repeatedly effective. When the data from the different animals were pooled, idiosyncratic variations in correct responding as a function of stimulus eccentricity were smoothed, but the multiplicative nature of the multisensory enhancement was still quite obvious.

Spatially Disparate Trials

In this situation animals were trained to respond only to the visual stimulus, which was made readily detectable by raising its intensity. During the training period responses to the auditory stimulus were never rewarded, and eventually the animals never responded to it. When the auditory stimulus came on during testing, it was simultaneous with the visual but was always 60 degrees away (figure 11.4). Now the probability of correctly responding to the visual stimulus declined dramatically. This is apparent in the example provided in figure 11.5. While the animals often failed to respond in any overt fashion, on many occasions they moved directly to a position halfway between the visual and the auditory stimuli, as if the neural integration of the two cues produced a phantom stimulus, one with no real physical counterpart.

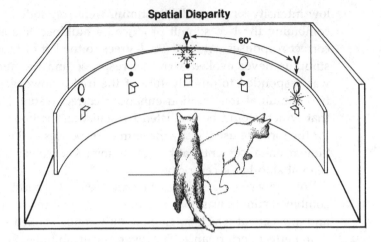

Spatial Disparity

Figure 11.4 Behavioral paradigm for studying the consequences of spatially disparate multisensory stimuli. Animals were trained to approach a visual stimulus but to ignore an auditory stimulus. During testing, the visual stimulus was presented alone (e.g., 60°) or in combination with an auditory stimulus that was 60° out of register with it (e.g., auditory at 0°, visual at 60°). The intensity of the visual stimulus was set so that a high percentage of correct responses were elicited to it alone. (From Stein et al. 1989)

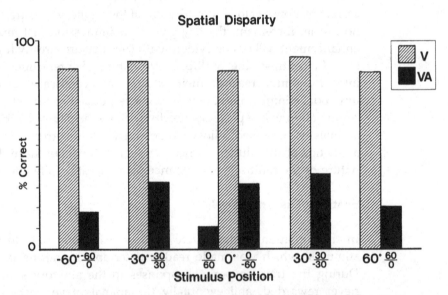

Figure 11.5 Spatially disparate stimuli depress correct responding. A visual (V) stimulus was presented at each of five locations. It was also presented in combination with an auditory stimulus (AV) 60° out of register with it. Although the animal never responded to the disparate auditory stimulus, it depressed responses to the visual stimulus. (From Stein et al. 1989)

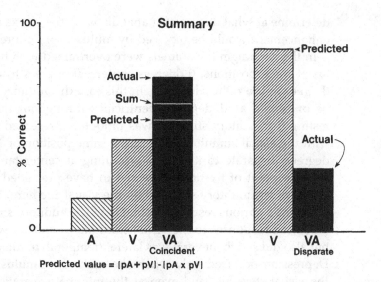

Figure 11.6 Summary: varying visual-auditory spatial relationships. In the spatially coincident paradigm, the enhancement produced in all cats (n = 4) significantly (p < 0.001) exceeded statistical predictions (formula at bottom) as well as the sum of the responses to unimodal auditory and visual stimuli. When the auditory and visual stimuli were combined in the spatially disparate paradigm (60° disparity), correct responses were markedly reduced (p < 0.001). (From Stein et al. 1989)

Stimulus intensity was as critical here as in the spatially coincident tests: high-intensity visual stimuli were responded to very well, even in the presence of a spatially disparate auditory stimulus. Regardless of the paradigm, highly effective stimuli that command an animal's attention are difficult to enhance or degrade with innocuous cues from other modalities. This is not only consistent with the electrophysiological observations, but is intuitively obvious as well.

A summary figure (figure 11.6), in which spatial coincidence and spatial disparity data were combined for all animals, illustrates the general behavioral results of these experiments. Pairing the stimuli at the same location facilitated detection and orientation performance that exceeded the predicted score, and even the sum of scores in response to the stimuli when presented individually. Similarly, the depressive effects of a disparate auditory stimulus were evident despite the fact that the animals were either trained to ignore it, or had no experience with it during training.

Spatial Resolution Trials

The spatial resolution paradigm was initiated to deal with two additional issues. First, results of the electrophysiological experiments indicated that an auditory stimulus should be effective even if the animals were not exposed to it during training, and we wanted to know if this would indeed be the case behaviorally. Second, it was of interest to determine at what degree of spatial disparity the effects of multisensory enhancement would be replaced by multisensory depression.

In this paradigm the animals were overtrained with the visual stimulus at three positions: 0 degrees center, 30 degrees to the left, and 30 degrees to the right. However, in this case the auditory stimulus could be presented at 15-degree eccentricities throughout the field. During testing the auditory stimulus was randomly presented simultaneously with the visual stimulus either at the same position or 15, 30, 45, or 60 degrees disparate to it. The overtraining at center target (which was also the point of fixation) appeared to have precluded any modifying effects of the auditory stimulus on the visual cue here, but at the other positions a curious result was obtained. The auditory stimulus not only enhanced responses to the visual stimulus when they were coincident, but also did so whenever it was lateral (temporal) to the visual stimulus. Depression occurred only when the auditory stimulus was medial to the visual stimulus, and even at the minimal separation used (15 degrees), as shown in figure 11.7.

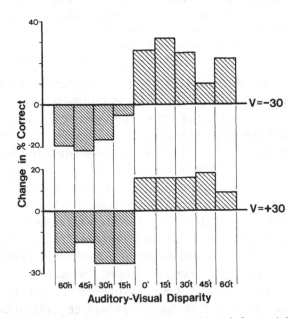

Figure 11.7 Relative location, not relative disparity, initiates behavioral depression. Animals (n = 3) were trained to approach a visual stimulus at 30°left ($-30°$) or right ($+30°$), but to ignore any auditory stimulus. During testing the visual stimulus was presented alone or in combination with an auditory stimulus coincident with it (0°), or 15°, 30°, 45°, or 60° disparate to it (either nasal, n; or temporal, t). The differences in responses to the visual alone and each combination are plotted. Note the response enhancements when the auditory stimulus was coincident with the visual at 30° left or right (i.e., 0° disparity) or when the auditory stimulus was temporal to it. In contrast, response depression occurred when the auditory stimulus was nasal to the visual. (Redrawn from Stein et al. 1989)

Multisensory Convergence and Integration at the Level of the Single Neuron

Overall, these behavioral data appear to be very similar to those generated in electrophysiological experiments: spatially coincident stimuli produce response enhancement (with enhancements being multiplicative and greatest with low-intensity stimuli), and spatially disparate stimuli produce either response depression or no apparent interaction. This makes sense because of the spatial register of multisensory receptive fields. But despite these observations, a simple transfer of this rule from the single neuron level to predicting the behavioral consequences of multisensory stimuli in space is not accurate unless the entire population of activated neurons is considered. The clearest evidence of this is the observation (see Spatial Resolution Trials) that an auditory stimulus temporal (and thus disparate) to a visual stimulus enhances orientation, and one medial to it (also disparate) depresses orientation. How could this happen if spatial coincidence = enhancement, and spatial disparity = depression?

Although this result seems to contradict the multisensory relationships established at the single neuron level, it is actually consistent with it, as shown in figure 11.8. Many auditory receptive fields that include temporal space are large, with medial borders 20–30 degrees from midline and lateral borders extending 120–180 degrees into peripheral space. Consequently, a temporal (>30 degrees) auditory stimulus is likely to enhance the physiological effects of a visual stimulus at 30 degrees peripheral because it falls into excitatory regions of most auditory receptive fields here. On the other hand, many of these same receptive fields have inhibitory medial borders. A stimulus even slightly medial to 30 degrees should encroach on these regions and inhibit the physiological effects of the visual stimulus.

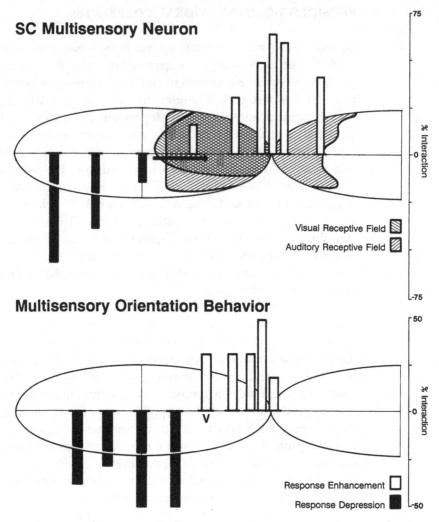

SC Multisensory Neuron

Visual Receptive Field
Auditory Receptive Field

% Interaction

Multisensory Orientation Behavior

V

Response Enhancement
Response Depression

% Interaction

Figure 11.8 Neuronal and behavioral similarities. The response interactions of a characteristic multisensory neuron are shown at the *top*. When an auditory stimulus is coincident with or temporal to the visual stimulus (arrow), enhancement is produced. This is because the posterior borders of the auditory receptive field reach far into temporal space. In contrast, nasal auditory stimuli fall beyond the medial border of the auditory receptive field and produce response depression. The same effect is obtained behaviorally (*bottom*; V refers to the position of the LED). Behavioral results are likely due to the similar distribution of populations of multisensory receptive fields.

The Importance of Topographic Register

MAINTAINING ALIGNMENT OF SENSORY MAPS

Because the receptive fields of unimodal neurons in each modality in the superior colliculus are large, a small eye (or ear, or body) movement has little effect on the alignment of the different sensory maps. Perhaps, during the course of evolution, large receptive fields were selected and maintained in multisensory structures as a way of offsetting the disruptive influences that small misalignments of sensory organs would have on multisensory register. If so, one would expect that animals with little or no independent mobility of peripheral sensory organs would not have been subjected to such pressures. After all, if they couldn't move their sensory organs relative to one another, they couldn't misalign multisensory receptive fields. Such animals would be better off developing the greater spatial resolution that accompanies small receptive fields.

This appears to have been the case for visual-auditory neurons in the optic tectum of the barn owl, an animal largely incapable of disrupting visual-auditory multisensory register because it has neither mobile ears nor the capacity for making eye movements of any significant magnitude. Instead, it shifts its eyes and ears in concert by moving its head (Knudsen 1982). Although this still allows some disruption of multisensory register with the rest of the body, the major tactile organ (the head) remains in register with the eyes and ears. The small receptive fields of owl tectal neurons contrast sharply with those of neurons in the superior colliculus of cat, ferret, and primate, species that exhibit a wide range of independent eye and ear movements (Gordon 1973; King and Hutchings 1987; Middlebrooks and Knudsen 1984; Jay and Sparks 1984, 1987b; Meredith and Stein 1986b, 1990).

The owl appears to be more the exception than the rule, and because it is so unusual to find a higher vertebrate that lacks the capability of independent eye movements, incredulity is generally the first reaction upon learning that an owl has to move its head to look around. This is because, unlike amphibians (Werner and Himstedt 1985), most higher vertebrates have the capability for impressively large independent eye movements and often possess mobile ears as well. In general, their range of eye and ear (and limb) movements is so great that there is little difficulty in significantly misaligning the peripheral sensory organs so that the register among the different receptive fields of many multisensory neurons would be significantly degraded. Combinations of stimuli that are coincident in space might then no longer fall within the respective receptive fields of the same multisensory neurons and produce response depression rather than enhancement. This would compromise the animal's detection and localization capabilities—a seemingly unavoidable consequence of an animal selectively scanning its surroundings with one set of peripheral sensors.

The mechanism for this disruptive effect is explained below, using an example in which a large eye movement is made while the head and ears remain in their initial positions. Since most animals frequently use eye movements to scan their environments, it is perhaps the most common instance of peripheral sensory organ misalignments. The effect of eye movements on multisensory alignment is similar for both superior colliculi, but for simplicity, only the left (contralateral) superior colliculus will be used in this example.

Because the visual map in the superior colliculus is really a map of the retinas, moving the eyes (and thus the retinas) produces a shift in the area of the superior colliculus activated by a stimulus fixed in space. Imagine a typical cartoon sequence, in which a small yellow bird with a speech impediment is making some moral point or other. The cat is looking straight ahead at the bird. He is attempting to suppress a normal cat's reaction because he notices the ear of a large dog that Grandma has assigned as "bird protector." The bird is seen and heard by the cat nearly simultaneously. The stimulus produces a focus of activity in the same position in the visual and auditory maps, as well as enhanced activity in many multisensory neurons there. The focus of activity corresponds to a rostral locus in the (left) superior colliculus, because it is here that visual and auditory receptive fields representing central space are found. If, however, instead of looking straight ahead, the cat's eyes were turned far to the left (a posture calculated to convince the now glaring dog that he really has no interest in this particular pedantic bird), the image of the bird will fall on other parts of the cat's retinas. Now the same stimulus produces visually evoked activity further caudal in the cat's superior colliculus, where those regions of the retinas (i.e., temporal visual space) are represented. But the bird's verbal staccato should still activate rostral superior colliculus: the bird didn't budge, only the cat's eyes shifted. The result, illustrated in figure 12.1, is that movement of the eyes caused a misalignment of visual and nonvisual maps, producing discordant sites of activation in the superior colliculus.

In this example, there is little doubt that the cat knows exactly where the bird is and can easily deal with him if only the dog would leave for a minute. The stimulus is extremely strong, all modalities are fully

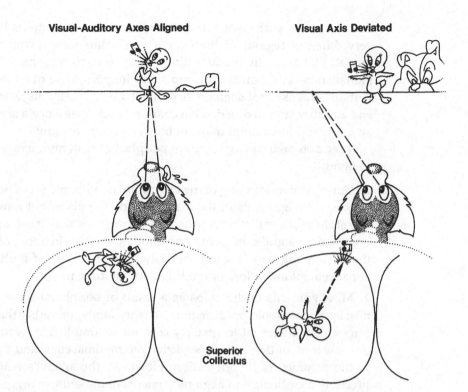

Visual-Auditory Axes Aligned **Visual Axis Deviated**

Superior
Colliculus

Figure 12.1 A paradox: Are representations of multisensory stimuli dissociated when the
visual and auditory axes are misaligned? When the cat's visual and auditory axes are
aligned, the representation of the image and sound of the bird are coincident in the
superior colliculus. However, when the presence of the dog induces the cat to shift his
gaze away from the bird, the visual image of the bird falls on a part of the cat's retina
which is mapped further posterior in the superior colliculus. Since the cat's ears and head
did not move, one would expect that the auditory representation of the bird remains at
the same, anterior location.

activated, and multisensory enhancement is of little importance. In non-
cartoon circumstances, however, when sensory cues may be minimal
and the cat is very real and very hungry, misaligments in the maps
could have disastrous consequences if there were no compensatory
mechanisms to deal with it. For it is precisely during hunting (as well
as predator avoidance) that minimal cues are of major significance for
survival, and that multisensory integration has its maximal effects on
enhancing meaningful stimuli and screening potential distractors. Undoubtedly the "hunting stance" facilitates integration and detection of
minimal cues by aligning all sensory organs and pointing them all in
the direction of potential prey. However, in circumstances in which
there is misalignment of the maps, the different receptive fields of multisensory neurons will also be misaligned, the enhancing potential of
these neurons to spatially coincident stimuli may be eliminated, or even
converted to inhibition, and detection of prey would be compromised.
Furthermore, if the different sensory inputs retain some of their effec-

tiveness under such circumstances, they will activate outputs from two very different regions of the superior colliculus (one rostral and one caudal) that normally produce different orientation responses. Their simultaneous activation would lead to an inappropriate overt response, perhaps one like that sometimes produced by spatially disparate visual and auditory stimuli described in chapter 11 (also see Kurylo et al. 1989): an orientation to a point midway between the two stimuli.

Three potential consequences of peripheral organ misalignment come to mind:

1. During active scanning of the environment with one set of peripheral organs, misalignments of the maps would take place, but a functional decoupling of conflicting sensory inputs ensures that these inputs do not interfere significantly with one another. In this situation, of course, the decoupling would simultaneously produce a loss of multisensory enhancement and a loss of multisensory inhibition.

2. Misalignments of the maps as a result of peripheral sensory organ misalignment would produce multisensory inhibition rather than multisensory enhancement to spatially coincident stimuli. This would result in a lowering of the animal's sensitivity to minimal cues, and a decrease in the accuracy of its orientation. However, the animal's tendency to precisely coordinate and align movements of the sensory organs in situations of focused attention, and/or heightened alertness, would avoid this problem when sensitivity and coordinated responses are most important.

3. Movement of one set of sensory organs would produce compensatory shifts of the other sensory maps in the superior colliculus, so that map alignment is maintained even though the peripheral organs are misaligned.

So far there is no empirical support for the first possible form of compensation, in which there is a decoupling of sensory systems. In fact, passively moving one set of sensory organs in anesthetized cats misaligns the receptive fields of multisensory neurons, as shown in chapter 10. Yet, the spatial rule of multisensory integration is not suppressed (i.e, decoupled) by the misalignment. Rather, stimuli coincident in space now produce response depression rather than response enhancement because one of the stimuli falls outside its excitatory receptive field and into the inhibitory portion of its receptive field (see figure 10.10). Such a finding is consistent with the second scenario presented above, and one would predict that not only would enhanced sensitivity to low-intensity multisensory cues fail to be produced, but sensitivity would decrease below that present for each cue individually.

To examine whether or not this lowered sensitivity actually occurs in a behaving animal, we have tried using a slight modification of the behavioral paradigms described in chapter 11. Cats are trained to fixate their eyes at 15 degrees to the right, rather than at 0 degrees (the choice of 15 degrees was made because the behavioral experiments described earlier showed that this was the minimal visual-auditory spatial disparity in which depression might occur). Because their heads and ears are pointed straight ahead, this fixation point should produce a significant misalignment of the eyes and ears, and presumably a misalignment of the maps of visual and auditory space in the brain. However, while the animals are willing to make a 15-degree saccade, they are very reluctant to maintain their eyes in that position even for several seconds, and even after thousands of trials none of our cats will maintain eccentric fixation long enough to test the postulate. They will move their eyes briefly to the right, but will follow with a head movement or shift their eyes back to 0 degrees almost immediately. Undoubtedly, a more sophisticated training paradigm or a greater incentive will prove successful in training cats to maintain large eccentric fixations for longer periods, but the repeated failures indicate that they just don't like to do this, at least not in our situation, in which the correct detection of low-intensity sensory stimuli will provide them with a significant reward. It is difficult to avoid concluding that the animals have learned to maximize their sensitivities to environmental events by maintaining alignment of their peripheral sensory organs. This would also be consistent with the second possibility raised above.

Observations in primates are consistent with the third possibility. In a very clever series of experiments, Jay and Sparks (1984, 1987a) have shown that when the rhesus monkey moves its eyes but keeps its head and ears in their original positions, the effective site of an auditory stimulus for activating a superior colliculus neuron is altered in a compensatory fashion. For example, an auditory stimulus that was effective in activating a neuron when the eyes were in what is called *primary orbital position* (looking straight ahead) lost much of its effectiveness when the eyes moved to the right. A new effective auditory locus now appeared to the right of the original site, as shown in figure 12.2.

The explanation offered for this shift in the position of an effective auditory stimulus is a parsimonious one. The different sensory maps are coded in motor-error coordinates, rather than in orbital or head coordinates: they code the motor-error signal (i.e., the trajectory and amplitude of the eye movement) that is necessary to visually fixate the target. Thus, the auditory map in the primate is assumed to be linked to eye movements just as is the visual map. Indeed, many of the same neurons exhibit presaccadic bursts to either auditory or visual targets (Jay and Sparks 1987b). The hypothesis also assumes that there is actually a map of auditory space in the primate superior colliculus like the one described in the cat. Although neither auditory nor somatosensory maps have been described in the primate superior colliculus, the assumption of an auditory map seems warranted, not only on the basis of the map in cat, but because effective auditory stimuli for the multisen-

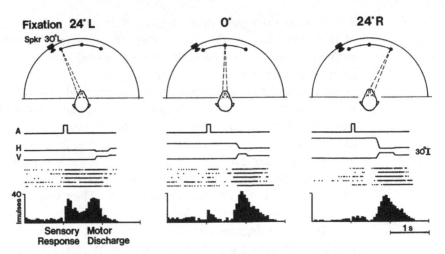

Figure 12.2 The auditory receptive field in a primate shifts with eye position. The schematics at the top indicate eye position (fixations are at 24° left, center, and 24° right) in relation to the location of the auditory stimulus (30° left). The top three traces in each panel represent the auditory stimulus (A), horizontal (H; up = rightward) and vertical (V; up = upward) eye position traces. After the onset of the auditory stimulus, eye movements were made to acquire it. Rasters show the activity of a superior colliculus neuron during five trials and are above cumulative histograms for the same trials. The initial sensory response is clearly affected by eye position, as it decreases with the difference between initial eye position and the target. (Redrawn from Jay and Sparks 1987b)

sory neurons in the monkey superior colliculus that have been studied are in rough topographic register with their visual receptive fields just as in the cat. Somatosensory-responsive neurons are also present in the primate superior colliculus (Berman and Cynader 1972), although their topography has not yet been detailed. It also remains to be seen in monkeys whether the effective site of a somatosensory stimulus exhibits spatial shifts with eye movements, as in the auditory representation.

The compensatory auditory shifts that have been observed in the primate are not complete, and the average shift of the effective auditory stimulus in space was about half that of the eye movement that initiated it. Since the entire auditory receptive field was not generally mapped, especially the temporal border (a rather difficult thing to do in the short period of time that the monkey maintains its eyes in the eccentric position), it is not clear whether the major shift in sensitivity is due to a mobile best area within the field. This possibility would explain the limitations of any shift: it could not exceed the actual borders of the auditory receptive field. Consistent with this possibility are observations in which stimulation within the original locus becomes less effective but still has the ability to evoke some activity (see figure 12.2). On the other hand, there were cases in which the temporal border was shown to shift with eye movements. These observations are consistent with a shift of the entire receptive field. Yet regardless of whether the best area of the receptive field or the receptive field itself moves, the result is a functional shift of auditory sensitivity.

While it is tempting to generalize directly from the observations made in behaving monkeys to all other animals (especially those that are visually dominant), there are some obvious hazards in doing so. Although Harris and colleagues (1980) examined only a limited sample of neurons in the alert cat, they noted that eye position did not influence the auditory responses of superior colliculus neurons in this animal. Furthermore, even if one applies the motor-error hypothesis across species, it is not immediately obvious that motor-error signals relate only to the eye movement. This is especially true in animals with mobile ears (or other mobile sensory organs). Movements of the external ears can shift auditory receptive fields (Middlebrooks and Knudsen 1987; figure 12.3; also see figure 10.10) and can thus shift the map of auditory space. If the locations of auditory receptive fields were to be tied only to eye movements, as suggested by observations in primates, the observed shifts of auditory receptive fields with ear movements in cats should not occur when the referent eye position is unchanged. Because the

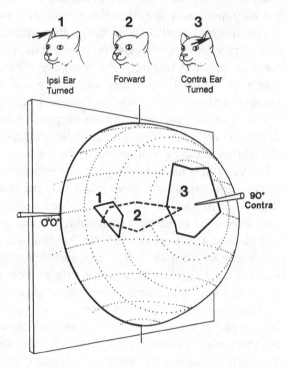

Figure 12.3 Changes in ear position shifts auditory receptive fields. The cat sits in the center of the sphere with its nose directed at the 0°,0° point (where the plane bisects auditory space; only the contralateral field is shown). Plotted is the best area of a superior colliculus auditory receptive field (2) when the ears are in normal forward position. The best area shifts frontally (1) with backward shifts of the ipsilateral ear, or laterally (3) with a backward shift of the contralateral ear. (Modified from Middlebrooks and Knudsen 1987)

The Importance of Topographic Register

ears shift to fixate an auditory target much like the eyes shift to fixate a visual target, it would be interesting to determine if ear movement (or limb movement) premotor neurons are present in the superior colliculus of any species to initiate these movements. If so, it would make little sense to shift the map of auditory space to coincide with the altered visual map, as the auditory map would then be out of register with its own ear movement map.

Whether or not there prove to be species differences in terms of the mobility of the different maps, or the strategies used to keep them aligned during overt behavior, the key feature for multisensory integration is the maintenance of sensory register itself. From a functional perspective it is less important *how* this is accomplished than the fact *that* it is accomplished, and thus far all the observations are consistent with a maintained spatial register among maps by one means or another.

DEVELOPING ALIGNMENT OF SENSORY MAPS

The fact that the various maps in the superior colliculus actually develop the alignment and spatial register with one another that is so crucial for meaningful multisensory integration appears to be more than just serendipity. Active processes operate to ensure that multisensory alignment is achieved during early ontogeny. This is evident from experiments in which the sensory experiences of developing animals are manipulated to produce aberrant sensory representations.

Raising a barn owl with one ear plugged changes the relative weights of the binaural cues that are used to construct its auditory map (i.e., the relative timing and intensity of inputs to the two ears). A maximally effective plug is likely to eliminate the effectiveness of the ear for all but the loudest sounds and leave intact only the comparatively weak inputs derived from bone conduction. Such an animal must learn to function on the basis of these abnormal binaural cues: a very strong input from one ear and a very weak one from the other ear even when the stimulus is directly in front of it. Yet, the auditory map that develops in such ear-occluded animals is in surprisingly good register with the visual map, and both maps *seem* quite normal (Knudsen 1982, 1983).

Apparently, some process that matches visual and auditory inputs is operative during early development and ensures that the visual and auditory maps eventually overlap each other regardless of the fact that the auditory inputs are atypical. Consequently, multisensory neurons develop receptive fields that are in spatial register with one another, just as in normally reared animals; an example of this is shown in figure 12.4. It appears that in the formation of the auditory map the nervous system looks to the visual map for alignment cues and uses these to determine the weighting or balance of inputs from the two ears. If the ear plug is removed when the animal becomes an adult, the input from

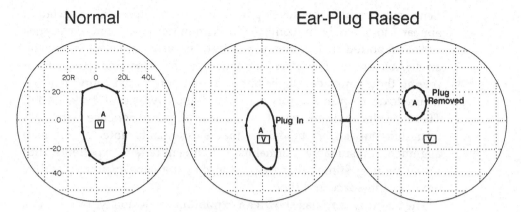

Figure 12.4 Normal auditory-visual register develops in owl optic tectum even when one ear is occluded. The auditory and visual receptive fields are closely aligned in bimodal neurons of normal owls (*left*, from Knudsen 1982 by permission of the *Journal of Neuroscience*) and owls raised with a sound-attenuating plug in one ear (*center*, from Knudsen 1983). However, if this plug is removed as an adult, the auditory field shifts and becomes misaligned with the visual (*right*, from Knudsen, E. I. (1983). Early auditory experience aligns the auditory map of space in the optic tectum of the barn owl. *Science* 222: 939–942)

the previously deprived ear is far stronger than it was when the auditory map was first formed and stabilized. The initial computation is now "incorrect" and the auditory map is shifted and displaced relative to the unaltered visual map (figure 12.4). It seems rather odd that correcting the developmental anomaly of a poorly functioning ear results in a dysfunction, misaligning the visual and auditory maps. But once the sensitive period for map stabilization is over, the "correction" is really a disruption of the compensation that aligned the auditory map with the visual map in the first place. The preeminence of the visual input in this animal is evident not only from these experiments, but also from experiments in which the visual input is displaced during early development by ocular prisms. Now the animal's auditory localization shifts toward the perceived (and incorrect) visual location of the target (Knudsen and Knudsen 1989b).

The capacity to develop aligned visual-auditory maps in the presence of atypical visual or auditory experience is by no means restricted to the owl or even to birds; it appears to be equally effective in mammals. King and co-workers (1988) have shown that an effect similar to the one described in the owl can be obtained in ferrets that have had one ear occluded or one eye deviated. In both cases a shift in the best area of auditory receptive fields was noted so that a functional compensation took place to align visual and auditory representations. If it is the experience with visual and auditory cues that dictates whether or not map alignment will occur, rather than the exact positions and relationships of the eyes and ears in the head during development, one would expect that eliminating the possibility of the visual-auditory multisensory experience will preclude the development of aligned maps. This expectation appears to have been confirmed. Withington-Wray and colleagues (1990a) reported that guinea pigs raised in darkness failed to develop an auditory map. Therefore, no alignment of maps took place. Even rearing these animals in light but with omnidirectional sound led to a failure to develop an auditory map (Withington-Wray et al. 1989, 1990b). These results indicate that it is not the simple experience with cues from different sensory modalities that is essential for intersensory map alignment. Presumably, normal map alignment reflects experience with visual-auditory stimuli that are produced by the same event so that they are linked in space and time.

The auditory map has shown an extraordinary flexibility. But even its flexibility is limited to a certain age and magnitude of displacement. Prism-induced compensation must occur during early development and even if produced during early maturation in owl, for example, adjustments of sound localization can be no greater than about 20 degrees (Knudsen and Knudsen 1989). Similarly, while ocular deviations of 15–20 degrees produce compensatory shifts in the auditory map in developing ferrets, a far greater displacement of the visual map, such as that produced by rotation of the eye, cannot be compensated for, and results in a rather disordered auditory representation (King et al. 1988).

The stability of the visual map contrasts sharply with the flexibility of the auditory map. In the face of a radically altered sensory environment, the visual map remains remarkably unmoved. Perhaps this is because the visual map is a direct, albeit somewhat distorted, reflection of the peripheral receptor surface rather than a derived, or computational, construct. If this is the reason, one would expect there to be no effect of peculiar visual and/or auditory rearing conditions on the somatotopic map, for it, too, is a direct (although geometrically distorted) reflection of the receptor surface. Unfortunately, the effects on somatotopic organization of altering visual and/or auditory inputs have not yet been evaluated in behaving animals; however, the data that are available from anesthetized animals indicate that, in contrast to the auditory map, the somatotopy (like the visuotopy) lacks topographic flexibility. In addition, Harris (1982) found that the somatosensory map in anophthalmic salamanders was normal and was unaffected by the orientation of the visual map that resulted from transplanting eyes in these animals. Furthermore, Rhoades (1980) and Rhoades et al. (1981) have noted that in hamsters, anomalies in the visual map induced by unilateral enucleation can also result in some anomalies in the receptive field properties of somatosensory neurons, but do not substantially alter the somatotopic map. Even the mirror-symmetric visual map produced by removal of the contralateral eye and contralateral superior colliculus in neonatal hamsters (forcing the ipsilateral eye to project to the remaining superior colliculus) does not result in a realignment of the somatosensory map (Mooney et al. 1987). As in the case of unilateral enucleation, this dramatic change in the visual map has effects on many somatosensory receptive field properties (e.g., they become larger, many become bilateral or exhibit split areas of sensitivity), but not enough of an effect on the arrangement of receptive fields to induce a mirror-symmetric topography that would match the visuotopy.

There is no doubt that mechanisms exist for guiding "corrective" changes during development within and across sensory maps. There is also no doubt that these mechanisms did not evolve in anticipation of the surgical manipulations that neuroscientists would perform. The purpose of flexibility in *within*-map construction during early ontogeny is, in part, to deal with the continuous developmental changes that occur, such as the separation between the eyes and ears and the gradual growth of the various peripheral sensory organs. In order to maintain alignment *among* maps it is most parsimonious to use one referent scheme, or map, to which other sensory maps are aligned. The data indicate that the stable referent, at least for the auditory system, is the visual map. This observation emphasizes the developmental importance of the visual system and would have fit nicely with Apter's intuition, nearly half a century ago, that the retinotopy is the basis for some organizational calibration in the superior colliculus.

The situation with the somatotopy is less clear. Some receptive field changes do occur with changes in the visuotopy, but the map itself appears to be quite stable. Perhaps the formation of the somatotopy is largely independent of pertubations in the other maps because, unlike the auditory and visual systems, the somatosensory system does not deal with stimuli in extrapersonal space and cannot compensate for changes in the sensory systems that do. Therefore, it follows its own developmental sequence. Fortunately, this is not usually a problem. The computational nature of the auditory map makes it so flexible that if there are slight physical differences that produce misalignments in the axes of the eyes and ears, they are readily compensated for. This ensures visual-auditory register in the brain and, unless these peripheral misalignments are extraordinarily large, the overlapping visual and auditory maps will also be in register with the somatosensory map.

13 Are the Rules of Multisensory Integration the Same in Different Areas of the Central Nervous System?

The alignment of the different sensory representations in the brain, and the alignment-maintenance system (or systems) that operates during overt behavior to preserve multisensory register, most likely evolved because alignment proved to be a critical feature of multisensory integration. Presumably, anything that facilitates map alignment and multisensory integration also facilitates detection, orientation, and perception and is likely to be selected and preserved in speciation. Therefore, one would expect that areas other than the superior colliculus in which multiple sensory inputs are found would have spatially aligned sensory maps, and that the same spatial and temporal rules of multisensory integration operating in superior colliculus neurons would apply to multisensory neurons found in these areas.

THE ALIGNMENT OF MULTISENSORY RECEPTIVE FIELDS

Comparatively little information is available about how the different receptive fields of multisensory neurons, outside the superior colliculus, relate to one another. Nevertheless, observations in several areas, including those in primary sensory cortices, are consistent with the idea that the spatial register of multisensory receptive fields is a generalized phenomenon.

For some reason, during the 1960s and 1970s a number of studies were designed with the apparent intention of demonstrating that "visual" cortex was not really the exclusive domain of the visual system. Many of these were successful, showing that activity could be evoked in visual cortical neurons by electrically shocking the forepaws, inducing pain with cutaneous pinpricks, or by presenting any of a wide variety of frequency-specific or broadband auditory stimuli (e.g., Lomo and Mollica 1962; Jung et al. 1963; Murata et al. 1965; Horn 1965; Spinelli et al. 1968; Morrell 1972; Fishman and Michael 1973). Even discounting the instances in which the stimuli probably produced activity via a general arousal influence, there were sufficient observations to demonstrate that at least some visual cortical neurons are responsive to nonvisual inputs and are thus multisensory.

Fishman and Michael (1973) noted that there were a number of visual-auditory neurons in visual cortical areas 17 and 18 of the cat. With only a few exceptions the auditory stimulus was effective only when it was placed in the same location in space as the visual receptive field. Morrell (1972) made similar observations in cat cortex. He found visual-auditory neurons in areas 18 and 19, and examined their sensitivities to stimulus position by presenting the same visual and auditory stimuli at each of a number of points equally spaced along the horizontal meridian. He reported that bimodal neurons responded to auditory and visual stimuli at the same points along this axis. A given neuron even preferred movements in the same directions in the different modalities. In at least one example, moving a visual stimulus opposite to the direction preferred or placing it in the inhibitory region of the visual receptive field not only inhibited spontaneous activity, but inhibited the response to an auditory stimulus as well.

The receptive fields of multisensory neurons have also been identified in the intraparietal and temporal cortices of rhesus monkey (Hikosaka et al. 1988; Duhamel et al. 1991). There, too, a close correspondence between their different sensory receptive fields exists, although some exceptions have been noted. Typically, however, a bimodal visual-somatosensory neuron with its visual receptive field in upper visual space has its somatosensory receptive field on the head, while more temporal visual receptive fields are found in neurons that have somatosensory receptive fields on the side of the head and shoulder—a relationship quite similar to that seen in the superior colliculus. The same sort of topographic register is seen in all modality combinations.

MULTISENSORY INTEGRATION IN CORTEX

Recently, we have begun examining the organization of multisensory neurons in the cortex of the cat, specifically the anterior ectosylvian sulcus (AES) and the dorsal bank of the most rostral portions of the lateral suprasylvian sulcus (LS), both of which are association cortices. As described earlier, the AES has a representation of the body surface (somatosensory area 4, or SIV) in its rostral aspect, a visual representation (anterior ectosylvian visual area, or AEV) caudal and ventral to SIV, and an auditory representation (Field AES) in its most caudal aspect. Distributed near the borders between these areas are multisensory neurons. All of these multisensory neurons that have been studied so far have receptive fields with the same kinds of cross-modal spatial registers as described for multisensory neurons in the superior colliculus, which is particularly noteworthy, since of all the sensory representations in the AES, only SIV has a sensory map (see Clemo and Stein 1982, 1983). The other sensory representations in AES lack an overall spatiotopic organization (Mucke et al. 1982; Olson and Graybiel 1987; Clarey and Irvine 1990). There must be something quite special about

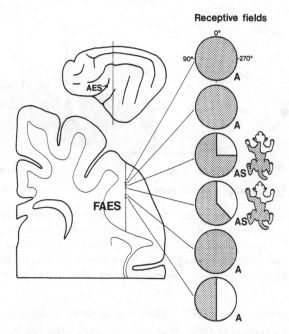

Receptive fields

Figure 13.1 Multisensory receptive field register in cortex. Neurons in the caudal portion of the anterior ectosylvian sulcal cortex (FAES) respond primarily to auditory stimuli. When the auditory receptive fields are mapped along a recording penetration, no auditory spatiotopic organization is apparent. However, the auditory (A) and somatosensory (S) receptive fields of neighboring bimodal neurons do exhibit close spatial register.

these multisensory neurons for them to match the spatial locations of their various sensory receptive fields (figure 13.1).

The only thing "quite special" that seemed likely to set these neurons apart from their unimodal counterparts is that, like multisensory neurons in the superior colliculus, their task is to integrate different sensory inputs. If such integration is to be meaningful, the relationships between modalities in these particular cortical neurons cannot be random, regardless of the organization of their nearest unimodal neighbors. In light of what we know about superior colliculus neurons, it was likely that the spatial coincidence of these neurons was a reflection of their multisensory integrative capabilities. To examine this possibility, the same paradigms of spatial and temporal tests that had been used to study superior colliculus neurons were used to study AES neurons (Wallace et al. 1992).

The results obtained so far are, indeed, quite similar to those obtained in multisensory superior colliculus neurons. For example, in a visual-auditory neuron (figure 13.2), the two receptive fields overlap in contralateral space. When the visual and auditory stimuli were presented in combination and within their respective receptive fields, the neuron's response was significantly better than that evoked by either stimulus alone. Using the formula described in chapter 10, the enhancement

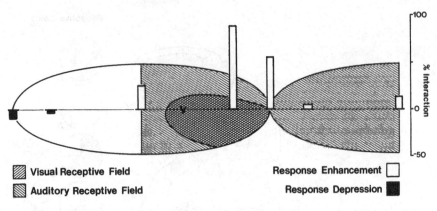

□ Visual Receptive Field

▨ Auditory Receptive Field

Response Enhancement □

Response Depression ■

Figure 13.2 The spatial rule of multisensory integration applies to cortex. The site of the visual stimulus was fixed at V. Its combination with an auditory stimulus at seven different locations (bars) evoked dramatically different response interactions. When the stimuli were within their receptive fields, response enhancement occurred; however, when the auditory stimulus was presented outside its receptive field, response depression resulted.

proved to be 88%. When the auditory stimulus was presented outside its receptive field, it minimally degraded the effectiveness of the visual stimulus. Furthermore, presenting the auditory stimulus far enough out of temporal synchrony with the visual stimulus also resulted in a depression of the visual response. Similar tests on somatosensory-auditory neurons yielded similar results. In one example the somatosensory and auditory receptive fields were both extraordinarily large. When spatially coincident contralateral auditory and somatosensory stimuli were combined, the response was significantly enhanced. However, when the auditory stimulus was presented in ipsilateral auditory space, the response to the somatosensory stimulus was significantly depressed.

The same findings are being obtained in multisensory neurons located in the multisensory (i.e., far rostral) region of LS. Here, too, we noted that the different receptive fields of a multisensory neuron overlap one another, the spatial and temporal rules of multisensory integration are operative, and in both areas the greatest multisensory enhancements were obtained with the weakest unimodal stimuli (Stein et al. 1993). Furthermore, unimodal receptive field properties appear unchanged in the presence of another sensory stimulus, even when the second stimulus substantially changes the neuron's overall level of responsiveness to the first.

CONCLUDING REMARKS

The observations described here strongly suggest that the spatial register among the receptive fields of multisensory neurons and their temporal response properties provide a neural substrate for enhancing responses to stimuli that covary in space and time and for degrading responses that are not spatially and temporally related. In other words, a neural mechanism exists by which the detection of minimal but meaningful stimulus combinations are facilitated and distracting stimuli are screened. It is quite likely that during early development the correlated multisensory activity in these neurons produces the close alignment of their receptive fields, which forms a key feature of multisensory integration in adults. In the case of the superior colliculus, multisensory neurons constitute the bulk of the neurons in each individual map. Therefore, their receptive field alignment produces alignment among all the maps.

The importance of map alignment for survival helps explain the extraordinary lengths to which the nervous systems of animals as diverse as fishes, reptiles, birds, and mammals have gone to develop and maintain spatial register among sensory representations in the midbrain. The mechanism itself is ancient, and its retention in a wide variety of species indicates its broad applicability in very different environmental circumstances. We now know that the alignment of different sensory maps is not unique to the superior colliculus, or even to the midbrain, but is a fundamental property of multisensory neurons in diverse structures and species.

While the rules that govern the synthesis of visual, auditory, and somatosensory cues appear to be similar throughout the brain, the results of these similar processes in different structures must surely have very different impacts on behavior and perception. We know very little about this at the moment. It should be quite evident that what has been learned thus far about the neural bases of pooling information from different sensory systems represents only a beginning.

An enormous number of challenges must be met before we understand more fully the processes involved in integrating information from different sensory modalities shown schematically in figure 13.3. We must learn not only how the consequences of this integration differ depending on the specific circuits activated, but how the integration of different sensory cues has been adapted to best serve the needs of different species; how membrane and subcellular mechanisms make it work; and what the rules of integration are among sensory modalities other than visual, auditory, and somatosensory (e.g., chemical senses). It is also an opportune time to begin combining noninvasive physiological techniques with perceptual evaluations in human subjects (see Hillyard et al. 1984; Costin et al. 1991). The technical advances in such physiological measures as event-related potentials, positron emission tomography and magnetic resonance imaging make it possible to apply what has been learned from physiological and behavioral studies in animals to studies of human subjects. By doing so, these observations will be extended not only directly to ourselves, undoubtedly the most interesting of all species, but also to the experiential and affective consequences of this form of integration. This strategy will enable us to take aim at one

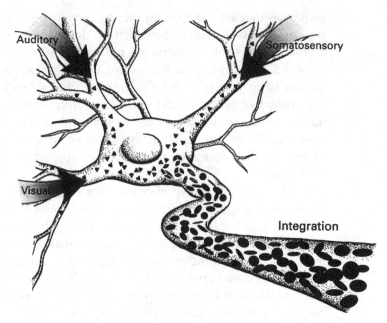

Figure 13.3 Neurons synthesize information from different sensory modalities.

of the primary goals of sensory physiology: a better understanding of the relationship between physiological processes and perceptual experiences. Despite the loftiness of this goal, the reality is that far too many details about how "simpler," within-modality information coding affects behavior and perception still remain elusive. Unraveling the mysteries of integration across multiple modalities will require even greater effort. In anticipation of the struggles ahead for those who would address some of these questions, perhaps there is some comfort in the remark made not long ago by a noted neuroscientist at a meeting, "It is better not to understand something complex, than not to understand something simple."

One final thought. In the Introduction we alluded to the aesthetic involved in the study of sensory systems. On reflection, it seems curiously appropriate that beauty is a characteristic of the very systems from which aesthetic appreciation is derived. For this attribute is not intrinsic to the objects, but, as most eloquently stated by David Hume, it is an attribute of the "mind which contemplates them." This contemplation, which involves sensory integration, is directed toward the creation of a harmonious synthesis, and as such perhaps represents the most satisfying product of a merging of the senses.

References

Abravanel, E. (1981) Integrating the information from eyes and hands. In *Intersensory Perception and Sensory Integration*, R. D. Walk and L. H. Pick, Jr. (eds.). New York: Plenum, pp. 71–108.

Ackerman, D. (1990) *A Natural History of the Senses*. New York: Vintage Books/Random House.

Adamuk, E. (1870) Uber die Innervation der Augenbewegungen. Zentralbl. Med. Wiss. 8:65–67.

Albano, J. E., Mishkin, M., Westbrook, L. E. and Wurtz, R. H. (1982) Visuomotor deficits following ablation of monkey superior colliculus. J. Neurophysiol. 48:338–351.

Alkon, D. L. (1983) Learning in a marine snail. Sci. Am. 249:70–84.

Altman, J. and Malis, L. I. (1962) An electrophysiological study of the superior colliculus and visual cortex. Exp. Neurol. 5:233–249.

Altner, H., Loftus, R., Schaller-Selzer, L. and Tichy, H. (1983) Modality-specificity in insect sensilla and multimodal input from body appendages. In *Multimodal Convergence in Sensory Systems*, E. Horn (ed.). New York: Fisher Verlag, pp. 17–32.

Amassian, V. E. and Devito, R. V. (1954) Unit activity in the reticular formation and nearby structures. J. Neurophysiol. 17:575–603.

Anderson, F. D. and Berry, C. M. (1959) Degeneration studies of long ascending fiber systems in the cat brain stem. J. Comp. Neurol. 3:195–229.

Anderson, P. A. V. and Mackie, G. O. (1977) Electrically coupled, photosensitive neurons control swimming in a jellyfish. Science 197:186–188.

Anderson, P. A. V. and Schwab, W. E. (1982) Recent advances and model systems in coelenterate neurobiology. Prog. Neurobiol. 19:213–236.

Andreassi, J. L. and Greco, J. R. (1975) Effects of bisensory stimulation on reaction time and the evoked cortical potential. Physiol. Psychol. 3:189–194.

Anisfeld, M., Masters, J. C., Jacobson, S. W. and Kagan, J. (1979) Interpreting "imitative" responses in early infancy. Science 205:214–219.

Apter, J. T. (1945) Projection of the retina on the superior colliculus of cats. J. Neurophysiol. 8:123–134.

Apter, J. T. (1946) Eye movements following strychninization of the superior colliculus of cats. J. Neurophysiol. 9:73–86.

Archer, P. W., Meredith, M. A. and Stein, B. E. (1990) Neurons in posterior cerebellum of rat respond to somatosensory and auditory stimuli. Soc. Neurosci. Abstr. 16:893.

Aronson, E. and Rosenbloom, S. (1971) Space perception in early infancy: Perception within a common auditory-visual space. Science 172:1161–1163.

Asanuma, C., Ohkawa, R., Stanfield, B. B. and Cowan, W. M. (1988) Observations on the development of certain ascending inputs to the thalamus in rats. I. Postnatal development. Dev. Brain Res. 41:159–170.

Astruc, J. (1971) Corticofugal connections of area 8 (frontal eye field) in *Macaca mulatta*. Brain Res. 161:241–256.

Atweh, S. F., Banna, N. R., Jabbur, S. J. and Tomey, G. G. (1974) Polysensory interactions in the cuneate nucleus. J. Physiol. 238:343–355.

Auroy, P., Irthum, B. and Woda, A. (1991) Oral nociceptive activity in the rat superior colliculus. Brain Res. 549:275–284.

Avanzini, G., Spreafico, R., Broggi, G., Giovannini, P. and Franceschetti, S. (1977) Topographic distribution of visual and somesthesic unitary responses in the Pul-LP complex of the cat. Neurosci. Lett. 4:135–143.

Azizi, S. A. and Woodward, D. J. (1990) Interactions of visual and auditory mossy fiber input in the paraflocculus of the rat: A gating action of multimodal inputs. Brain Res. 533:255–262.

Baleydier, C., Kahungu, M. and Mauguiere, F. (1983) A crossed corticotectal projection from the lateral suprasylvian area in the cat. J. Comp. Neurol. 214:344–351.

Ballam, G. O. (1982) Bilateral and multimodal sensory interactions of single cells in the pigeon's midbrain. Brain Res. 245:27–35.

Barasi, S. (1979) Responses of substantia nigra neurones to noxious stimulation. Brain Res. 171:121–130.

Bartels, M., Munz, H. and Claas, B. (1990) Representation of lateral line and electrosensory systems in the midbrain of the axolotl, *Ambystoma mexicanum*. J. Comp. Physiol. [A] 167:347–356.

Bastian, J. (1982) Vision and electroreception: Integration of sensory information in the optic tectum of the weakly electric fish *Apteronotus albifrons*. J. Comp. Physiol. 147:287–297.

Bauer, U. and Hatt, H. (1980) Demonstration of three different types of chemosensitive units in the crayfish claw using a computerized evaluation. Neurosci. Lett. 208–214.

Beckstead, R. M. (1979) An autoradiographic examination of corticocortical and subcortical projections of the mediodorsal-projection (prefrontal) cortex in the rat. J. Comp. Neurol. 184:43–62.

Beckstead, R. M. and Frankfurter, A. (1983) A direct projection from the retina to the intermediate gray layer of the superior colliculus demonstrated by anterograde transport of horseradish peroxidase in monkey, cat and rat. Exp. Brain Res. 52:261–268.

Behan, M. and Appell, P. P. (1992) Intrinsic circuitry in the cat superior colliculus: Projections from the superficial layers. J. Comp. Neurol. 315:230–243.

Behan, M., Appell, P. P. and Graper, M. J. (1988) Ultrastructural study of large efferent neurons in the superior colliculus of the cat after retrograde labeling with horseradish peroxidase. J. Comp. Neurol. 270:171–184.

Bell, C., Sierra, B., Buendia, N. and Segundo, J. P. (1964) Sensory properties of neurons in the mesencephalic reticular formation. J. Neurophysiol. 27:961–987.

Benevento, L. A., Fallon, J. H., Davis, B. and Rezak, M. (1977) Auditory-visual interaction in single cells in the cortex of the superior temporal sulcus and the orbital frontal cortex of the macaque monkey. Exp. Neurol. 57:849–872.

Berman, N. and Cynader, M. (1972) Comparison of receptive-field organization of the superior colliculus in Siamese and normal cats. J. Physiol. (Lond.) 224:363–389.

Bernstein, I. H. (1970) Can we see and hear at the same time? Acta Psychol. 33:21–35.

Bernstein, I. H., Clark, M. H. and Edelstein, B. A. (1969) Effects of an auditory signal on visual reaction time. J. Exp. Psychol. 80:567–569.

Berson, D. M. (1985) Cat lateral suprasylvian cortex: Y-cell inputs and corticotectal projections. J. Neurophysiol. 53:544–556.

Berson, D. M. and McIlwain, J. T. (1982) Retinal Y-cell activation of deep-layer cells in superior colliculus of the cat. J. Neurophysiol. 47:700–714.

Berthoz, A. and Jones, G. M. (1985) *Reviews of Oculomotor Research, Volume I: Adaptive Mechanisms in Gaze Control.* New York: Elsevier.

Berthoz, A., Grantyn, A. and Droulez, J. (1986) Some collicular efferent neurons code saccadic eye velocity. Neurosci. Lett. 72:294–298.

Biguer, B., Donaldson, I. M. L., Hein, A. and Jeannerod, M. (1988) Neck muscle vibration modifies the representation of visual motion and direction in man. Brain 111:1405–1424.

Blomqvist, A., Flink, R., Bowsher, D., Griph, S. and Westman, J. (1978) Tectal and thalamic projections of dorsal column and lateral cervical nucleus: A quantitative study in the cat. Brain Res. 141:335–341.

Bodznick, D. (1991) Elasmobranch vision: Multimodal integration in the brain. J. Exp. Zool. Suppl. 5:108–116.

Bower, T. G. R. (1974) The evolution of sensory systems. In *Perception: Essays in Honor of James J. Gibson*, R. G. MacLeod and H. L. Pick, Jr. (eds.). Ithaca: Cornell University Press, pp. 141–165.

Bower, T. G. R. (1977) *A Primer of Infant Development.* San Francisco: W. H. Freeman.

Bower, T. G. R., Broughton, J. M. and Moore, M. K. (1970) The coordination of visual and tactual input in infants. Perception and Psychophysics 8:51–53.

Boyd, A. and Simon, M. (1982) Bacterial chemotaxis. Annu. Rev. Physiol. 44:501–517.

Bruce, C., Desimone, R. and Gross, C. G. (1981) Visual properties of neurons in a polysensory area in superior temporal sulcus of the macaque. J. Neurophysiol. 46:369–384.

Bruce, L. L., McHaffie, J. G. and Stein, B. E. (1987) The organization of trigeminotectal and trigeminothalamic neurons in rodents: A double-labeling study with fluorescent dyes. J. Comp. Neurol. 262:315–330.

Buisseret, P. and Maffei, L. (1983) Suppression of visual cortical activity following tactile periorbital stimulation: Its role during eye blinks. Exp. Brain Res. 51:463–466.

Bullock, T. H. (1984) Physiology of the tectum mesencephali in elasmobranchs. In *Comparative Neurology of the Optic Tectum*, H. Vanegas (ed.). New York: Plenum, pp. 47–68.

Burgess, P. R. (1973) Cutaneous mechanoreceptors. In *Handbook of Perception*, E. C. Carterette and M. P. Friedman (eds.). New York: Academic, pp. 219–249.

Burton, H., Mitchell, G. and Brent, D. (1982) Second somatic sensory area in the cerebral cortex of cats: Somatotopic organization and cytoarchitecture. J. Comp. Neurol. 210: 109–135.

Butterworth, G. (1981) The origins of auditory-visual perception and visual proprioception in human development. In *Intersensory Perception and Sensory Integration*, R. D. Walk and L. H. Pick, Jr. (eds.). New York: Plenum, pp. 37–70.

Caan, W., Delgado-Garcia, J., Stein, J. F. and Watam-Bell, J. (1976) Interaction of visual and auditory inputs to the cerebellar Purkinje cells in cat posterior vermis. J. Physiol. (Lond.) 258:20P-21P.

Campion, J., Latto, R. and Smith, Y. M. (1983) Is blindsight an effect of scattered light, spared cortex, and near-threshold vision? Behav. Brain Sci. 6:423–486.

Casagrande, V. A., Harting, J. K., Hall, W. C. and Diamond, I. T. (1972) Superior colliculus of the tree shrew: A structural and functional subdivision into superficial and deep layers. Science 177:444–447.

Caston, J. and Bricout-Berthout, A. (1984) Responses to somatosensory input by afferent and efferent neurons in the vestibular nerve of the frog. Brain Behav. Evol. 24: 135–143.

Caston, J. and Bricout-Berthout, A. (1985) Influence of stimulation of the visual system on the activity of vestibular nuclear neurons in the frog. Brain Behav. Evol. 26:49–57.

Cazin, L., Precht, W. and Lannou, J. (1980) Optokinetic responses of vestibular nucleus neurons in the rat. Pfluger Arch. 384:31–38.

Chalupa, L. M. and Fish, S. E. (1978) Response characteristics of visual and extravisual neurons in the pulvinar and lateral posterior nuclei of the cat. Exp. Neurol. 61:96–120.

Chalupa, L. M. and Rhoades, R. W. (1977) Responses of visual, somatosensory, and auditory neurones in the golden hamster's superior colliculus. J. Physiol. (Lond.) 207:595–626.

Chalupa, L. M., Macadar, A. W. and Lindsley, D. B. (1975) Response plasticity of lateral geniculate neurons during and after pairing of auditory and visual stimuli. Science 190:290–292.

Chapman, C. E., Spadalieri, G. and Lamarre, Y. (1986) Activity of dentate neurons during arm movements triggered by visual, auditory, and somesthetic stimuli in the monkey. J. Neurophysiol. 55:203–226.

Chevalier, G. and Deniau, J. M. (1987) The striato-nigro-collicular pathway: A route for facial information to oculo and cephalic motor circuits. In *Basal Ganglia and Behavior: Sensory Aspects of Motor Functioning*, J. S. Schneider and T. I. Lidsky (eds.). Toronto: Hans Huber, pp. 83–88.

Chevalier, G., Vacher, S. and Deniau, J. M. (1984) Inhibitory nigral influence on tectospinal neurons, a possible implication of basal ganglia in orienting behavior. Exp. Brain Res. 53:320–326.

Clarey, J. C. and Irvine, D. R. F. (1986) Auditory response properties of neurons in the anterior ectosylvian sulcus of the cat. Brain Res. 386:12–19.

Clarey, J. C. and Irvine, D. R. F. (1990) The anterior ectosylvian sulcal auditory field in the cat: I. An electrophysiological study of its relationship to surrounding auditory cortical fields. J. Comp. Neurol. 301:289–303.

Clark, B. and Graybiel, A. (1966) Contributing factors in the perception of the oculogravic illusion. Am. J. Psychol. 79:377–388.

Clemo, H. R. and Stein, B. E. (1982) Somatosensory cortex: A "new" somatotopic representation. Brain Res. 235:162–168.

Clemo, H. R. and Stein, B. E. (1983) Organization of a fourth somatosensory area of cortex in cat. J. Neurophysiol. 50:910–925.

Clemo, H. R. and Stein, B. E. (1984) Topographic organization of somatosensory corticotectal influences in cat. J. Neurophysiol. 51:843–858.

Clemo, H. R. and Stein, B. E. (1986) Effects of cooling somatosensory cortex on response properties of tactile cells in the superior colliculus. J. Neurophysiol. 55:1352–1368.

Clemo, H. R. and Stein, B. E. (1987) Responses to direction of stimulus movement are different for somatosensory and visual cells in cat superior colliculus. Brain Res. 405: 313–319.

Clemo, H. R. and Stein, B. E. (1991) Internal organization of somatosensory receptive fields in the cat superior colliculus. J. Comp. Neurol. 314:534–544.

Clemo, H. R., Meredith, M. A., Wallace, M. T. and Stein, B. E. (1991) Is the cortex of cat anterior ectosylvian sulcus a polysensory area? Soc. Neurosci. Abstr. 17:1585.

Cohen, B. (ed.) (1981) *Vestibular and Oculomotor Physiology: International Meeting of the Barany Society.* Annals of the New York Academy of Sciences, Vol. 374.

Cohen, B. and Henn, V. (eds.) (1988) *Representation of Three-Dimensional Space in the Vestibular, Oculomotor, and Visual Systems.* Annals of the New York Academy of Sciences, Vol. 545.

Cohen, M. M. (1981) Visual-proprioceptive interactions. In *Intersensory Perception and Sensory Integration,* R. D. Walk and L. H. Pick, Jr. (eds.). New York: Plenum, pp. 175–314.

Colavita, R. B. (1974) Human sensory dominance. Percept. Psychophys. 16:409–412.

Colavita, R. B. and Weisberg, D. (1979) A further investigation of visual dominance. Percept. Psychophys. 25:345–357.

Collewijn, H. (1977) Gaze in freely moving subjects. In *Control of Gaze by Brain Stem Neurons. Developments in Neuroscience, Volume 1,* R. Baker and A. Berthoz (eds.). Amsterdam: Elsevier, pp. 13–22.

Comer, C., and Grobstein, P. (1981) Involvement of midbrain structures in tactually and visually elicited prey acquisition behavior in the frog *Rana pipiens.* J. Comp. Physiol. 142:151–160.

Costin, D., Neville, H. J., Meredith, M. A. and Stein, B. E. (1991) Rules of multisensory integration and attention: ERP and behavioral evidence in humans. Soc. Neurosci. Abstr. 17:656.

Cotter, J. R. (1976) Visual and nonvisual units recorded from the optic tectum of *Gallus domesticus.* Brain Behav. Evol. 13:1–21.

Coulter, J. D., Bowker, R. M., Wise, S. P., Murray, E. A., Castiglioni, A. J. and Westlund, K. N. (1979) Cortical, tectal and medullary descending pathways to the cervical spinal cord. Prog. Brain Res. 50:263–279.

Critchley, M. (1977) Ecstatic and synaesthetic experience during musical perception. In *Music and the Brain: Studies in the Neurology of Music,* M. Critchley and R. A. Henson (eds.). Springfield, Ill.: Charles C Thomas.

Crommelinck, M. and Roucoux, A. (1976) Characteristics of cat's eye saccades in different states of alertness. Brain Res. 103:574–578.

Cynader, M. and Berman, N. (1972) Receptive-field organization of monkey superior colliculus. J. Neurophysiol. 35:187–201.

Cytowic, R. E. (1989) *Synesthesia: A Union of the Senses.* New York: Springer-Verlag.

Dagan, D. and Parnas, I. (1970) Giant-fibre and small-fibre pathways involved in the evasive response of the cockroach, *Periplaneta americana.* J. Exp. Biol. 52:313–324.

Davis, H. (1968) Auditory responses evoked in the human cortex. In *Hearing Mechanisms in Vertebrates,* A. V. S. DeReuch and J. Knight (eds.). Boston: Little, Brown.

Dean, P. and Redgrave, P. (1984) The superior colliculus and visual neglect in rat and hamster. I. Behavioral evidence. Brain Res. Rev. 8:129–141.

Dean, P., Redgrave, P., Sahibzada, N. and Tsuji, K. (1986) Head and body movements produced by electrical stimulation of superior colliculus in rats: Effects of interruption of crossed tectoreticulospinal pathway. Neuroscience 19:367–380.

Dean, P., Mitchell, I. J. and Redgrave, P. (1988a) Contralateral head movements produced by microinjection of glutamate into superior colliculus: Evidence for mediation by multiple output pathways. Neuroscience 24:491–500.

Dean, P., Mitchell, I. J. and Redgrave, P. (1988b) Response resembling defensive behavior produced by microinjection of glutamate in superior colliculus of rats. Neuroscience 24:501–510.

De Ceccatty, M. P. (1974) The origin of the integrative systems: A change in view derived from research on coelenterates and sponges. Perspect. Biol. Med. 17:379–390.

Delgado, J. M. R. (1965) Cerebral structures involved in transmission and elaboration of noxious stimulation. J. Neurophysiol. 18:261–275.

de Peyer, J. and Machemer, H. (1978) Are receptor-activated ciliary motor responses mediated through voltage or current? Nature 276:285–287.

Diamond, I. T. (1967) The sensory neocortex. In *Contributions to Sensory Physiology, Volume 2*, W. D. Neff (ed.). New York: Academic Press, pp. 51–100.

Diamond, I. T. and Hall, W. C. (1969) Evolution of neocortex. Science 164:251–262.

Dichgans, J., Schmidt, C. L. and Graf, W. (1973) Visual input improves the speedometer function of the vestibular nuclei in the goldfish. Exp. Brain Res. 18:319–322.

Drager, U. C. and Hubel, D. H. (1975) Responses to visual stimulation and relationship between visual, auditory and somatosensory inputs in mouse superior colliculus. J. Neurophysiol. 38:690–713.

Drager, U. C. and Hubel, D. H. (1976) Topography of visual and somatosensory projections in mouse superior colliculus. J. Neurophysiol. 39:91–101.

Dubner, R. and Rutledge, L. T. (1964) Recording and analysis of converging input upon neurons in cat association cortex. J. Neurophysiol. 27:620–634.

Duhamel, J.-R., Colby, C. L. and Goldberg, M. E. (1991) Congruent representations of visual and somatosensory space in single neurons of monkey ventral intraparietal cortex (Area VIP). In *Brain and Space*, J. Paillard (ed.). New York: Oxford University Press, pp. 223–236.

Du Lac, S. and Knudsen, E. I. (1990) Neural maps of head movement vector and speed in the optic tectum of the barn owl. J. Neurophysiol. 63:131–146.

Ebbesson, S. O. E. (1980) Structure and connections of the optic tectum in elasmobranchs. In *Comparative Neurology of the Telencephalon*, S. O. E. Ebbesson (ed.). New York: Plenum, pp. 1–16.

Eckert, R. (1965) Bioelectric control of bioluminescence in the dinoflagellate *Noctiluca*. Science 147:1140–1145.

Eckert, R., Naitoh, Y. and Friedman, K. (1972) Sensory mechanisms in *Paramecium*. I. Two components of the electric response to mechanical stimulation of the anterior surface. J. Exp. Biol. 56:683–694.

Edwards, S. B. (1977) The commissural projection of the superior colliculus in the cat. J. Comp. Neurol. 173:23–40.

Edwards, S. B. (1980) The deep cell layers of the superior colliculus their reticular characteristics and structural organization. In *The Reticular Formation Revisited*, A. Hobson and M. A. Brazier (eds.). New York: Raven, pp. 193–209.

Edwards, S. B. and Henkel, C. K. (1978) Superior colliculus connections with the extraocular motor nuclei in the cat. J. Comp. Neurol. 179:451–468.

Edwards, S. B., Rosenquist, A. C. and Palmer, L. (1974) An autoradiographic study of the ventral lateral geniculate projections in the cat. Brain Res. 72:282–287.

Edwards, S. B., Ginsburgh, C. L., Henkel, C. K. and Stein, B. E. (1979) Sources of subcortical projections to the superior colliculus in the cat. J. Comp. Neurol. 184:309–330.

Ellard, C. G. and Goodale, M. A. (1986) The role of the predorsal bundle in head and body movements elicited by electrical stimulation of the superior colliculus in the Mongolian gerbil. Exp. Brain Res. 64:421–433.

Ellard, C. G. and Goodale, M. A. (1988) A functional analysis of the collicular output pathways: A dissociation of deficits following lesions of the dorsal tegmental decussation and the ipsilateral collicular efferent bundle in the Mongolian gerbil. Exp. Brain Res. 71:307–319.

Ettlinger, G. and Wilson, W. A. (1990) Cross-modal performance: Behavioural processes, phylogenetic considerations and neural mechanisms. Behav. Brain Res. 40:169–192.

Evinger, C. and Fuchs, A. F. (1978) Saccadic, smooth pursuit and optokinetic eye movements of the trained cat. J. Physiol. [Lond.] 285:209–229.

Ewert, J.-P. (1984) Tectal mechanisms that underlie prey-catching and avoidance behaviors in toads. In *Comparative Neurology of the Optic Tectum*, H. Vanegas (ed.). New York: Plenum.

Fallon, J. H. and Benevento, L. A. (1977) Auditory-visual interaction in cat orbital-insular cortex. Neurosci. Lett. 6:143–149.

Feldon, S., Feldon, P. and Kruger, L. (1970) Topography of the retinal projection upon the superior colliculus of the cat. Vision Res. 10:135–143.

Finkenstadt, T. and Ewert, J.-P. (1983) Visual pattern discrimination through interactions of neural networks: A combined electrical brain stimulation, brain lesion, and extracellular recording study in *Salamandra salamandra*. J. Comp. Physiol. 153:99–110.

Finlay, B. L., Schneps, S. E., Wilson, K. G. and Schneider, G. E. (1978) Topography of visual and somatosensory projections to the superior colliculus of the golden hamster. Brain Res. 142:223–235.

Fish, S. E. and Voneida, T. J. (1979) Extravisual neurons in the optic tectum of a sighted and an unsighted fish. Soc. Neurosci. Abstr. 5:784.

Fishman, M. C. and Michael, C. R. (1973) Integration of auditory information in the cat's visual cortex. Vision Res. 13:1415–1419.

Freeman, J. A. (1970) Responses of cat cerebellar Purkinje cells to convergent inputs from cerebral cortex and peripheral sensory systems. J. Neurophysiol. 33:697–712.

Frost, D. O. (1984) Axonal growth and target selection during development: retinal projections to the ventrobasal complex and other "nonvisual" structures in neonatal Syrian hamsters. J. Comp. Neurol. 230:576–592.

Gaither, N. S. and Stein, B. E. (1979) Reptiles and mammals use similar sensory organization in the midbrain. Science 205:595–597.

Gardner, J. and Gardner, H. (1970) A note on selective imitation by a six-week-old infant. Child Dev. 41:1209–1213.

Gazzaniga, M. S. (1988) Interhemispheric integration. In *Neurobiology of the Neocortex. The Dahlem Workshop*, P. Rakic (ed.). New York: John Wiley, pp. 385–405.

Gibson, E. J. (1983) The development of knowledge about intermodal unity: Two views. In *Piaget and the Foundation of Knowledge*, L. S. Lisben (ed.). Hillsdale, N.J.: Erlbaum.

Gibson, J. J. (1966) *The Senses Considered as Perceptual Systems*, Boston: Houghton Mifflin.

Gielen, S. C. A. M., Schmidt, R. A. and van den Heuvel, P. J. M. (1983) On the nature of intersensory facilitation of reaction time. Percept. Psychophys. 34:161–168.

Glezer, I. I., Jacobs, M. S. and Morgane, P. J. (1988) Implications of the "initial brain" concept for brain evolution in cetacea. Behav. Brain Sci. 11:75–116.

Goldberg, M. E. and Wurtz, R. H. (1972a) Activity of superior colliculus in behaving monkey. I. Visual receptive fields of single neurons. J. Neurophysiol. 35:542–559.

Goldberg, M. E. and Wurtz, R. H. (1972b) Activity of superior colliculus in behaving monkey. II. Effect of attention on neuronal responses. J. Neurophysiol. 35:560–574.

Goodale, M. (1973) Corticotectal and intertectal modulation of visual responses in the rat's superior colliculus. Exp. Brain Res. 17:75–86.

Goodale, M. A. and Murison, R. C. C. (1975) The effects of lesions of the superior colliculus on locomotor orientation and the orienting reflex in the rat. Brain Res. 88:243–261.

Gordon, B. G. (1973) Receptive fields in the deep layers of the cat superior colliculus. J. Neurophysiol. 36:157–178.

Gottlieb, G., Tomlinson, W. R. and Radell, P. L. (1989) Developmental intersensory interference: Premature visual experience suppresses auditory learning in ducklings. Infant Behav. Dev. 12:1–12.

Graeber, R. C. (1984) Behavioral correlates of tectal function in elasmobranchs. In *Comparative Neurology of the Optic Tectum*, H. Vanegas (ed.). New York: Plenum, pp. 69–90.

Graf, W., Simpson, I. and Leonard, C. (1988) Spatial organization of visual messages of the rabbit's cerebellar flocculus. II. Complex and simple spike responses of Purkinje cells. J. Neurophysiol. 60:2091–2121.

Graham, J. (1977) An autoradiographic study of the efferent connections of the superior colliculus in the cat. J. Comp. Neurol. 173:629–654.

Graham, J., Pearson, H. E., Berman, N. and Murphy, H. E. (1981) Laminar organization of superior colliculus in the rabbit: A study of receptive-field properties of single units. J. Neurophysiol. 45:915–932.

Grant, S. J., Aston-Jones, G. and Redmond, D. E. (1988) Responses of primate locus coeruleus neurons to simple and complex sensory stimuli. Brain Res. Bull. 21:401–410.

Grantyn, R. (1988) Gaze control through the superior colliculus: structure and function. In *Neuroanatomy of the Oculomotor System*, J. A. Buttner-Ennever (ed.). Amsterdam: Elsevier, pp. 273–333.

Grantyn, A. and Berthoz, A. (1985) Burst activity of identified tecto-reticulo-spinal neurons in the alert cat. Exp. Brain Res. 57:417–421.

Grantyn, A. and Grantyn, R. (1982) Axonal patterns and sites of termination of cat superior colliculus neurons projecting in the tecto-bulbo-spinal tract. Exp. Brain Res. 46: 243–265.

Graybiel, A. (1952) Oculogravic illusion. AMA Arch. Ophthalmol. 48:605–615.

Graybiel, A. and Niven, J. I. (1951) The effect of a change in direction of resultant force on sound localization: The audiogravic illusion. J. Exp. Psychol. 42:227–230.

Gregory, R. L. (1967) Origin of eyes and brains. Nature 213:369–372.

Grell, K. G. (1973) *Protozoology*. Berlin: Springer-Verlag.

Gruberg, E. R. and Solish, S. P. (1978) The relationship of a monoamine fiber system to a somatosensory tectal projection in the salamander, *Ambystoma tigrinum*. J. Morphol. 157:137–150.

Guitton, D. and Munoz, D. P. (1991) Control of orienting gaze shifts by the tectoreticulo-spinal system in the head-free cat. I. Identification, localization, and effects of behavior on sensory responses. J. Neurophysiol. 66:1605–1623.

Guitton, D., Crommelinck, M. and Roucoux, A. (1980) Stimulation of the superior colliculus in the alert cat. I. Eye movements and neck EMG activity evoked when the head is restrained. Exp. Brain Res. 39:63–73.

Guthrie, B. L., Porter, J. D. and Sparks, D. L. (1983) Corollary discharge provides accurate eye position information to the oculomotor system. Science 221:1193–1195.

Hardy, S. C. and Stein, B. E. (1988) Small lateral suprasylvian cortex lesions produce visual neglect and decreased visual activity in the superior colliculus. J. Comp. Neurol. 273:527–542.

Harris, L. R. (1980) The superior colliculus and movements of the head and eyes in cats. J. Physiol. 300:367–391.

Harris, L. R., Blakemore, C. and Donaghy, M. (1980) Integration of visual and auditory space in mammalian superior colliculus. Nature 288:56–59.

Harris, W. A. (1982) The transplantation of eyes to genetically eyeless salamanders: Visual projections and somatosensory interactions. J. Neurosci. 2:339–353.

Hartline, P. and Northmore, D. (1986) Precision of sound localization and coordination of eye and pinna movements by cats presented with visual and auditory targets. Soc. Neurosci. Abstr. 12:1277.

Hartline, P. H., Kass, L. and Loop, M. S. (1978) Merging of modalities in the optic tectum: Infrared and visual integration in rattlesnakes. Science 199:1225–1229.

Hartmann, R. and Klinke, R. (1980) Efferent activity in the goldfish vestibular nerve and its influence on afferent activity. Pflugers Arch. 388:123–128.

Hatt, H. (1986) Responses of a bimodal neuron (chemo- and vibration-sensitive) on the walking legs of the crayfish. J. Comp. Physiol. [A] 159:611–617.

Hatt, H. and Bauer, U. (1980) Single unit analysis of mechano- and chemosensitive neurones in the crayfish claw. Neurosci. Lett. 17: 203–207.

Heilingenberg, W. (1988) Electrosensory maps form a substrate for the distributed and parallel control of behavioral responses in weakly electric fish. Brain Behav. Evol. 31:6–16.

Held, R. (1955) Shifts in binaural localization after prolonged exposures to atypical combinations of stimuli. Am. J. Psychol. 68:526–548.

Helmholtz, H. von (1968) The origin of the correct interpretation of our sensory impressions. In *Helmholtz on Perception: Its Physiology and Development*, R. M. Warren and R. P. Warren (eds.). New York: Wiley, pp. 247–266.

Henn, V., Cohen, B. and Young, L. R. (1980) Visual-vestibular interaction in motion perception and the generation of nystagmus. Neurosci. Res. Prog. Bull. 18:459–651.

Hensler, K. (1989) Corrective flight steering in locusts: Convergence of extero- and proprioceptive inputs in descending deviation detectors. In *Neurobiology of Sensory Systems*, R. N. Singh and N. J. Strausfeld (eds.). New York: Plenum, pp. 531–554.

Henson, R. A. (1977) Neurological aspects of musical experience. In *Music and the Brain: Studies in the Neurology of Music*, M. Critchley and R. A. Henson (eds.). Springfield, IL: Charles C Thomas, pp. 3–21.

Herrick, C. J. (1948) *The Brain of the Tiger Salamander*. Chicago: University of Chicago Press.

Hershenson, M. (1962) Reaction time as a measure of intersensory facilitation. J. Exp. Psychol. 63:289–293.

Hicks, T. P., Benedek, G. and Thurlow, G. A. (1988) Modality specificity of neuronal responses within the cat's insula. J. Neurophysiol. 60:422–437.

Hikosaka, K., Iwai, E., Saito, H.-A. and Tanaka, K. (1988) Polysensory properties of neurons in the anterior bank of the caudal superior temporal sulcus of the macaque monkey. J. Neurophysiol. 60:1615–1637.

Hikosaka, O. and Wurtz, R. H. (1983) Visual and oculomotor functions of monkey substantia nigra pars reticulata. IV. Relation of substantia nigra to superior colliculus. J. Neurophysiol. 49:1285–1301.

Hikosaka, O. and Wurtz, R. H. (1985) Modification of saccadic eye movements by GABA-related substances. I. Effect of muscimol and bicuculline in monkey superior colliculus. J. Neurophysiol. 53:266–291.

Hikosaka, O., Sakamoto, M. and Usui, S. (1989) Functional properties of monkey caudate neurons II. Visual and auditory responses. J. Neurophysiol. 61:799–813.

Hille, B. (1984) *Ion Channels of Excitable Membranes*. Sunderland, Mass.: Sinauer Assoc. Inc.

Hille, B. (1989) Ionic channels: Evolutionary origins and modern roles. Quart. J. Exp. Physiol. 74:785–804.

Hillyard, S. A., Simpson, G. V., Woods, D. L., VanVoorhis, S. and Munte, T. F. (1984) Event-related brain potentials and selective attention to different modalities. In *Cortical Integration*, F. Reinoso-Suarez and C. Ajmone-Marsan (eds.). New. York: Raven, pp. 395–415.

Hirsch, J. A., Chan, C. K. and Yin, T. C. (1985) Responses of neurons in the cat's superior colliculus to acoustic stimuli. I. Monaural and binaural response properties. J. Neurophysiol. 53:726–745.

Hoffmann, K.-P. and Straschill, M. (1971) Influences of corticotectal and intertectal connections on visual responses in the cat's superior colliculus. Exp. Brain Res. 12:120–131.

Holcombe, V. and Hall, W. C. (1981) The laminar origin and distribution of the crossed tectoreticular pathways. J. Neurosci. 1:1103–1112.

Hooper, S. L. and Moulins, M. (1989) Switching of a neuron from one network to another by sensory-induced changes in membrane properties. Science 244:1587–1589.

Horn, E. (1983) *Multimodal Convergence in Sensory Systems*. Stuttgart: Gustav Fischer.

Horn, G. (1965) The effect of somaesthetic and photic stimuli on the activity of units in the striate cortex of unanesthetized, unrestrained cats. J. Physiol. 179:263–277.

Horn, G. and Hill, R. M. (1966) Responsiveness to sensory stimulation of units in the superior colliculus and subjacent tectotegmental regions of the rabbit. Exp. Neurol. 14:199–223.

Horn, K. M., Miller, S. W. and Neilson, H. C. (1983) Visual modulation of neuronal activity within the rat vestibular nuclei. Exp. Brain Res. 52:311–313.

Hotta, T. and Terashima, S. (1965) Audiovisual interaction and its correlation with cortical stimulation in the lateral thalamus. Exp. Neurol. 12:146–158.

Howard, I. P. and Templeton, W. B. (1966) *Human Spatial Orientation*. London: Wiley.

Huerta, M. F. and Harting, J. K. (1984a) Connectional organization of the superior colliculus. Trends Neurosci. 7:286–289.

Huerta, M. F. and Harting, J. K. (1984b) The mammalian superior colliculus: Studies of its morphology and connections. In *Comparative Neurology of the Optic Tectum*, H. Vanegas (ed.). New York: Plenum, pp.687–773.

Ingle, D. (1973a) Evolutionary perspectives on the function of the optic tectum. Brain Behav. Evol. 8:211–237.

Ingle, D. (1973b) Two visual systems in the frog. Science 181:1053–1055.

Innocenti, G. M. and Clarke, S. (1984) Bilateral transitory projection to visual areas from auditory cortex in kittens. Dev. Brain Res. 14:143–148.

Isaacson, R. L. (1987) Hippocampus. In *Encyclopedia of Neuroscience, Volume II*, G. Adelman (ed.). Boston: Birkhauser, pp. 492–495.

Itaya, S. K. and Van Hoesen, G. W. (1982) Retinal innervation of the inferior colliculus in rat and monkey. Brain Res. 233:45–52.

Ito, S.-I. (1982) Prefrontal unit activity of macaque monkeys during auditory and visual reaction time tasks. Brain Res. 247:39–47.

Jabbur, S. J., Atweh, S. F., Tomey, G. G. and Banna, N. R. (1971) Visual and auditory inputs into the cuneate nucleus. Science 174:1146–1147.

Jassik-Gerschenfeld, D. (1965) Somesthetic and visual responses of superior colliculus neurones. Nature 208:898–900.

Jassik-Gerschenfeld, D. and Hardy, O. (1984) The avian optic tectum: Neurophysiology and behavioral correlations. In *Comparative Neurology of the Optic Tectum*, H. Vanegas (ed.). New York: Plenum, pp. 649–686.

Jay, M. F. and Sparks, D. L. (1984) Auditory receptive fields in primate superior colliculus shift with changes in eye position. Nature 309:345–347.

Jay, M. F. and Sparks, D. L. (1987a) Sensorimotor integration in the primate superior colliculus. I. Motor convergence. J. Neurophysiol. 57:22–34.

Jay, M. F. and Sparks, D. L. (1987b) Sensorimotor integration in the primate superior colliculus. II. Coordinates of auditory signals. J. Neurophysiol. 57:35–55.

Jen, P. H., Sun, X., Kamada, T., Zhang, S. and Shimozawa, T. (1984) Auditory response properties and spatial response areas of superior collicular neurons in the FM bat, *Eptesicus fuscus*. J. Comp. Physiol. 154:407–413.

Jennings, H. S. (1906) *Behavior of Lower Animals*. Bloomington: Indiana University Press.

Jerison, H. J. (1973) *Evolution of the Brain and Intelligence*. New York: Academic Press.

Jones, B. (1981) The developmental significance of cross-modal matching. In *Intersensory Perception and Sensory Integration*, R. D. Walk and H. L. Pick (eds.). New York: Plenum, pp. 109–132.

Jones, E. G. and Powell, T. P. S. (1970) An anatomical study of converging sensory pathways within the cerebral cortex of the monkey. Brain 93:793–820.

Jung, R., Kornhuber, H. H. and Da Fonseca, J. S. (1963) Multisensory convergence on cortical neurons: neuronal effects of visual, acoustic and vestibular stimuli in the superior convolutions of the cat's cortex. In *Progress in Brain Research*, G. Moruzzi, A. Fessard and H. H. Jasper (eds.). Amsterdam: Elsevier, pp. 207–240.

Kaas, J. H. (1989) The evolution of complex sensory systems in mammals. J. Exp. Biol. 146:165–176.

Kanaseki, T. and Sprague, J. M. (1974) Anatomical organization of pretectal nuclei and tectal laminae in the cat. J. Comp. Neurol. 158:319–338.

Kao, C.-Q., McHaffie, J. G. and Stein, B. E. (1989) Response properties and somatotopy of vibrissa-activated neurons in rat superior colliculus. Soc. Neurosci. Abstr. 15:388.

Kao, C.-Q., McHaffie, J. G., Meredith, M. A., Clemo, H. R. and Stein, B. E. (1990) Comparative magnification of the vibrissa representation in the superior colliculus of rodents and cats. Soc. Neurosci. Abstr. 16:223.

Karabelas, A. B. and Moschovakis, A. K. (1985) Nigral inhibitory termination on efferent neurons of the superior colliculus: An intracellular horseradish peroxidase study in the cat. J. Comp. Neurol. 239:309–329.

Kawamura, K. and Hashikawa, T. (1978) Cell bodies of origin of reticular projections from the superior colliculus in the cat: An experimental study with the use of horseradish peroxidase as a tracer. J. Comp. Neurol. 182:1–16.

Kawamura, K. and Konno, T. (1979) Various types of corticotectal neurons of cats as demonstrated by means of retrograde axonal transport of horseradish peroxidase. Exp. Brain Res. 35:161–175.

Kawamura, S., Sprague, J. M. and Niimi, K. (1974) Corticofugal projection from the visual cortices to the thalamus, pretectum and superior colliculus in the cat. J. Comp. Neurol. 58:339–362.

Kawamura, S., Hattori, S., Higo, S. and Matsuyama, T. (1982) The cerebellar projections to the superior colliculus and pretectum in the cat: An autoradiographic and horseradish peroxidase study. Neuroscience 7:1673–1689.

Keay, K., Westby, G. W. M., Frankland, P., Dean, P. and Redgrave, P. (1990) Organization of the crossed tecto-reticulo-spinal projection in rat. II. Electrophysiological evidence for separate output channels to the periabducens area and caudal medulla. Neuroscience 37:585–601.

Keller, E. L. and Daniels, P. D. (1975) Oculomotor related interaction of vestibular and visual stimulation in vestibular nucleus cells in alert monkey. Exp. Neurol. 46:187–198.

Kenny, P. A. and Turkewitz, G. (1986) Effects of unusually early visual stimulation on the development of homing behavior in the rat pup. Dev. Psychobiol. 19:57–66.

King, A. J. and Hutchings, M. E. (1987) Spatial response properties of acoustically responsive neurons in the superior colliculus of the ferret: A map of auditory space. J. Neurophysiol. 57:596–624.

King, A. J. and Palmer, A. R. (1983) Cells responsive to free-field auditory stimuli in guinea-pig superior colliculus: Distribution and response properties. J. Physiol. 342: 361–381.

King, A. J. and Palmer, A. R. (1985) Integration of visual and auditory information in bimodal neurones in the guinea-pig superior colliculus. Exp. Brain Res. 60:492–500.

King, A. J., Hutchings, M. E., Moore, D. R. and Blakemore, C. (1988) Developmental plasticity in the visual and auditory representations in the mammalian superior colliculus. Nature 332:73–76.

Kluver, H. (1937) Certain effects of lesions of the occipital lobes in macaques. J. Psychol. 4:383–401.

Knudsen, E. I. (1982) Auditory and visual maps of space in the optic tectum of the owl. J. Neurosci. 2:1177–1194.

Knudsen, E. I. (1983) Early auditory experience aligns the auditory map of space in the optic tectum of the barn owl. Science 222:939–942.

Knudsen, E. I. and Brainard, M. S. (1991) Visual instruction of the neural map of auditory space in the developing optic tectum. Science 253:85–87.

Knudsen, E. I. and Knudsen, P. F. (1989) Vision calibrates sound localization in developing barn owls. J. Neurosci. 9:3306–3313.

Kohler, I. (1964) The formation and transformation of the perceptual world. Psychological Issues 3(4):1–173.

Koopowitz, H. (1975) Activity and habituation in the brain of the polyclad flatworm, *Freemania litoricola*. J. Exp. Biol. 62:455–467.

Krasne, F. B. (1965) Escape from recurring tactile stimulation in *Branchiomma vesiculosum*. J. Exp. Biol. 42:307–322.

Kruger, L. (1970) The topography of the visual projection to the mesencephalon: A comparative survey. Brain Behav. Evol. 3:169–177.

Kruger, L. and Stein, B. E. (1973) Primordial sense organs and the evolution of sensory systems. In *Handbook of Perception, Volume III*, E. C. Carterette and M. P. Friedman (eds.). New York: Academic, pp. 67–87.

Kung, C. and Saimi, Y. (1982) The physiological basis of taxes in *Paramecium*. Annu. Rev. Physiol. 44:519–534.

Kung, C., Saimi, Y. and Martinac, B. (1990) Mechano-sensitive ion channels in microbes and the early evolutionary origin of solvent sensing. In *Current Topics in Membranes and Transport, Volume 36*, J. F. Hoffman, G. Giebisch and T. Claudio (eds.), New York: Academic, pp. 145–153.

Kunzle, H. and Akert, K. (1977) Efferent connections of cortical area 8 (frontal eye field) in *Macaca fascicularis*. A reinvestigation using the autoradiographic technique. J. Comp. Neurol. 173:147–164.

Kurylo, D. D., Hartline, P. H. and Vimal, R. L. P. (1989) Effects of visual-auditory experience on saccadic localization of auditory stimuli. Soc. Neurosci. Abstr. 15:806.

Lackner, J. R. (1974a) Changes in auditory localization during body tilt. Acta Otolaryngol. (Stockh.) 19–28.

Lackner, J. R. (1974b) Influence of visual rearrangement and visual motion on sound localization. Neuropsychologia 12:291–293.

Land, M. F. and Fernald, R. D. (1992) The evolution of eyes. Annu. Rev. Neurosci. 15:1–29.

Larson, M. A., McHaffie, J. G. and Stein, B. E. (1987) Response properties of nociceptive and low-threshold mechanoreceptive neurons in the hamster superior colliculus. J. Neurosci. 7:547–564.

Lee, C., Rohrer, W. H. and Sparks, D. L. (1988) Population coding of saccadic eye movements by neurons in the superior colliculus. Nature 332:357–360.

Leichnetz, G. R., Spencer, R. F., Hardy, S. G. P. and Astruc, J. (1981) The prefrontal corticotectal projection in the monkey: An anterograde and retrograde horseradish peroxidase study. Neuroscience 6:1023–1041.

Leichnetz, G. R., Hardy, S. G. B. and Carruty, M. K. (1987) Frontal projections to the region of the oculomotor complex in the rat: A retrograde and anterograde HRP study. J. Comp. Neurol. 263:387–399.

Leonard, C. M. (1969) The prefrontal cortex of the rat. I. Cortical projections of the medio-dorsal nucleus. II. Efferent connections. Brain Res. 12:321–343.

Lickliter, R. (1990) Premature visual stimulation accelerates intersensory functioning in bobwhite quail neonates. Dev. Psychobiol. 23:15–27.

Lomo, T. and Mollica, A. (1962) Activity of single units in the primary optic cortex in the unanesthetized rabbit during visual, acoustic, olfactory and painful stimulation. Arch. Ital. Biol. 100:86–120.

Lyons-Ruth, K. (1977) Bimodal perception in infancy: Responses to auditory-visual incongruity. Child Dev. 48:820–827.

Ma, T. P., Cheng, H.-W., Czech, J. A. and Rafols, J. A. (1990) Intermediate and deep layers of the macaque superior colliculus: A Golgi study. J. Comp. Neurol. 295:92–110.

Mackie, G. O. and Passano, L. M. (1968) Epithelial conduction in hydromedusae. J. Gen. Physiol. 52:600–621.

Mackie, G. O. and Singla, C. L. (1983) Studies on hexactinellid sponges. I. Histology of *Rhabdocalyptus dawsoni* (Lamb, 1873). Phil. Trans. R. Soc. Lond. B301:365–400.

Marburg, O. and Warner, J. F. (1947) The pathways of the tectum (anterior colliculus) of the midbrain in cats. J. Nerv. Ment. Dis. 106:415–446.

Marks, L. E. (1975) On colored-hearing synesthesia: Cross-modal translations of sensory dimensions. Psychol. Bull. 82:303–331.

Marks, L. E. (1978) *The Unity of the Senses: Interrelations Among the Modalities.* New York: Academic.

Maronde, U. (1991) Common projection areas of antennal and visual pathways in the honeybee brain, *Apis mellifera.* J. Comp. Neurol. 309:328–340.

Martin, G. F. (1969) Efferent tectal pathways of the opossum *Didelphis virginiana.* J. Comp. Neurol. 135:209–224.

Mast, T. E. and Chung, D. Y. (1973) Binaural interactions in the superior colliculus of the chinchilla. Brain Res. 62:227–230.

Maunsell, J. H. R., Nealy, T. A., Sclar, G. and DePriest, D. D. (1989) Representation of extraretinal information in monkey visual cortex. In *Neural Mechanisms of Visual Perception. Proceedings of the Retina Research Foundation Symposia, Volume Two,* D. M.-K. Lam and C. D. Gilbert (eds.). Houston: Gulf Publishing, pp. 223–236.

Maurer, D. and Maurer, C. (1988) *The World of the Newborn.* New York: Basic Books.

May, P. J. and Porter, J. D. (1992) The laminar distribution of macaque tectobulbar and tectospinal neurons. Vis. Neurosci. 8:257–276.

May, P. J., Hartwich-Young, R., Nelson, J., Sparks, D. L. and Porter, J. D. (1990) Cerebro-tectal pathways in the macaque: Implications for collicular generation of saccades. Neuroscience 36:305–324.

Mays, L. E. and Sparks, D. L. (1980) Dissociation of visual and saccade-related responses in superior colliculus neurons. J. Neurophysiol. 43:207–232.

McGurk, H. and MacDonald, J. (1976) Hearing lips and seeing voices. Nature 264:746–748.

McHaffie, J. G. and Stein, B. E. (1981) Properties of cells activated by vibrissal movement in the superior colliculus of the rodent. Soc. Neurosci. Abstr. 7:393.

McHaffie, J. and Stein, B. E. (1982) Eye movements evoked by electrical stimulation in the superior colliculus of rats and hamsters. Brain Res. 247:243–253.

McHaffie, J. G., Kruger, L., Clemo, H. R. and Stein, B. E. (1988) Corticothalamic and corticotectal somatosensory projections from the anterior ectosylvian sulcus (SIV cortex) in neonatal cats: An anatomical demonstration with HRP and ^{3}H-leucine. J. Comp. Neurol. 274:115–126.

McHaffie, J. G., Kao, C.-Q. and Stein, B. E. (1989) Nociceptive neurons in rat superior colliculus: Response properties, topography, and functional implications. J. Neurophysiol. 62:510–525.

McHaffie, J. G., Norita, M., Dunning, D. D. and Stein, B. E. (1993) Corticotectal relationships: Direct and "indirect" corticotectal pathways. In *Progress in Brain Research: The Visually Responsive Neuron: From Basic Neurophysiology to Behavior*, T. P. Hicks, S. Molotchnikoff and T. Ono (eds.). Amsterdam: Elsevier, in press.

McIlwain, J. T. (1975) Visual receptive fields and their images in superior colliculus of the cat. J. Neurophysiol. 38:219–230.

McIlwain, J. T. (1986) Effects of eye position on saccades evoked electrically from the superior colliculus of alert cats. J. Neurophysiol. 55:97–112.

McIlwain, J. T. (1990) Topography of eye-position sensitivity of saccades evoked electrically from the cat's superior colliculus. Vis. Neurosci. 4:289–298.

McIlwain, J. T. (1991) Distributed spatial coding in the superior colliculus: A review. Visual Neurosci. 6:3–13.

Mehler, W. R., Feferman, M. E. and Nauta, W. J. H. (1960) Ascending axon degeneration following anterolateral cordotomy. An experimental study in the monkey. Brain 83: 718–752.

Meltzoff, A. N. (1990) Towards a developmental cognitive science: The implications of cross-modal matching and imitation for the development of representation and memory in infancy. Ann. N.Y. Acad. Sci. 608:1–37.

Meltzoff, A. N. and Kuhl, P. K. (1989) Infants' perception of faces and speech sounds: Challenges to developmental theory. In *Challenges to Developmental Paradigms*, P. R. Zelazo and R. G. Barr (eds.). Hillsdale, N.J.: Erlbaum, pp. 67–91.

Meltzoff, A. N. and Moore, M. K. (1977) Imitation of facial and manual gestures by human neonates. Science 198:75–78.

Meltzoff, A. N. and Moore, M. K. (1983a) The origins of imitation in infancy: Paradigm, phenomena, and theories. In *Advances in Infancy Research, Vol. 2*, L. P. Lipsitt (ed.). Norwood, N.J.: Ablex, pp. 265–301.

Meltzoff, A. N. and Moore, M. K. (1983b) Newborn infants imitate adult facial gestures. Child Dev. 54:702–709.

Meredith, M. A. and Clemo, H. R. (1989) Auditory cortical projection from the anterior ectosylvian sulcus (Field AES) to the superior colliculus in the cat: An anatomical and electrophysiological study. J. Comp. Neurol. 289:687–707.

Meredith, M. A. and Goldberg, S. J. (1986) Contractile differences between muscle units in the medial rectus and lateral rectus muscles in the cat. J. Neurophysiol. 56:50–62.

Meredith, M. A. and Stein, B. E. (1983) Interactions among converging sensory inputs in the superior colliculus. Science 221:389–391.

Meredith, M. A. and Stein, B. E. (1985) Descending efferents from the superior colliculus relay integrated multisensory information. Science 227:657–659.

Meredith, M. A. and Stein, B. E. (1986a) Visual, auditory, and somatosensory convergence on cells in superior colliculus results in multisensory integration. J. Neurophysiol. 56: 640–662.

Meredith, M. A. and Stein, B. E. (1986b) Spatial factors determine the activity of multisensory neurons in cat superior colliculus. Brain Res. 365:350–354.

Meredith, M. A. and Stein, B. E. (1990) The visuotopic component of the multisensory map in the deep laminae of the cat superior colliculus. J. Neurosci. 10:3727–3742.

Meredith, M. A., Nemitz, J. W. and Stein, B. E. (1987) Determinants of multisensory integration in superior colliculus neurons. I. Temporal factors. J. Neurosci. 10:3215–3229.

Meredith, M. A., Clemo, H. R. and Stein, B. E. (1991) Somatotopic component of the multisensory map in the deep laminae of the cat superior colliculus. J. Comp. Neurol. 312: 353–370.

Meredith, M. A., Wallace, M. T. and Stein, B. E. (1992) Visual, auditory and somatosensory convergence in output neurons of the cat superior colliculus: Multisensory properties of the tect-reticulo-spinal projection. Exp. Brain Res. 88:181–186.

Middlebrooks, J. C. (1987) Binaural mechanisms of spatial tuning in the cat's superior colliculus distinguished using monaural occlusion. J. Neurophysiol. 57:688–701.

Middlebrooks, J. C. and Knudsen, E. I. (1984) A neural code for auditory space in the cat's superior colliculus. J. Neurosci. 4:2621–2634.

Middlebrooks, J. C. and Knudsen, E. I. (1987) Changes in external ear position modify the spatial tuning of auditory units in the cat's superior colliculus. J. Neurophysiol. 57: 672–687.

Midgley, G. C., Wilkie, D. M. and Tees, R. C. (1988) Effects of superior colliculus lesions on rats' orienting and detection of neglected visual cues. Behav. Neurosci. 102:93–100.

Mistlin, A. J. and Perrett, D. I. (1990) Visual and somatosensory processing in the macaque temporal cortex: The role of "expectation." Exp. Brain Res 82:437–450.

Mize, R. R. (1983a) Patterns of convergence and divergence of retinal and cortical synaptic terminals in the cat superior colliculus. Exp. Brain Res. 51:88–96.

Mize, R. R. (1983b) Variations in the retinal synapses of the cat superior colliculus revealed using quantitative electron microscope autoradiography. Brain Res. 269:211–221.

Mohler, C. W. and Wurtz, R. H. (1976) Organization of monkey superior colliculus: Intermediate layer cells discharging before eye movements. J. Neurophysiol. 39:722–744.

Mooney, R. D., Klein, B. G., Jacquin, M. F. and Rhoades, R. W. (1984) Dendrites of deep layers, somatosensory superior collicular neurons extend into the superficial laminae. Brain Res. 324:361–365.

Mooney, R. D., Klein, B. G. and Rhoades, R. W. (1987) Effects of altered visual input upon the development of the visual and somatosensory representations in the hamster's superior colliculus. Neuroscience 20:537–555.

Mooney, R. D., Nikoletseas, M. M., Hess, P. R., Allen, Z., Lewin, A. C. and Rhoades, R. W. (1988) The projection from the superficial to the deep layers of the superior colliculus: An intracellular horseradish peroxidase injection study in the hamster. J. Neurosci. 8:1384–1399.

Mooney, R. D., Huang, X. and Rhoades, R. W. (1990) Effects of inactivation of the superficial laminae upon the visual responsivity of deep layer neurons in the hamster's superior colliculus. Soc. Neurosci. Abstr. 16:109.

Mori, A., Hanashima, N., Tsuboi, Y., Hiraba, H., Goto, N. and Sumino, R. (1991) Fifth somatosensory cortex (SV) representation of the whole body surface in the medial bank of the anterior suprasylvian sulcus of the cat. Neurosci. Res. 11:198–208.

Morrell, F. (1972) Visual system's view of acoustic space. Nature 238:44–46.

Morrell, L. K. (1968a) Cross-modality effects upon choice reaction time. Psychonom. Sci. 11:129–130.

Morrell, L. K. (1968b) Temporal characteristics of sensory interaction in choice reaction times. J. Exp. Psychol. 77:14–18.

Morris, C. E. (1990) Mechanosensitive ion channels. J. Membr. Biol. 113:97–107.

Moschovakis, A. K. and Karabelas, A. B. (1985) Observations on the somatodendritic morphology and axonal trajectory of intracellularly HRP-labeled efferent neurons located in the deeper layers of the superior colliculus of the cat. J. Comp. Neurol. 239:276–308.

Moschovakis, A. B., Karabelas, A. B. and Highstein, S. M. (1988a) Structure-function-relationships in the primate superior colliculus. I. Morphological classification of efferent neurons. J. Neurophysiol. 60:232–262.

Moschovakis, A. B., Karabelas, A. B. and Highstein, S. M. (1988b) Structure-function-relationships in the primate superior colliculus. II. Morphological identity of presaccadic neurons. J. Neurophysiol. 60:263–302.

Mucke, L., Norita, M., Benedek, G. and Creutzfeldt, O. (1982) Physiologic and anatomic investigation of a visual cortical area situated in the ventral bank of the anterior ectosylvian sulcus of the cat. Exp. Brain Res. 46:1–11.

Munoz, D. P. and Guitton, D. (1985) Tectospinal neurons in the cat have discharges coding gaze position error. Brain Res. 341:184–188.

Munoz, D. P. and Guitton, D. (1986) Effect of attention on tecto-reticulo-spinal neuron sensory and motor discharges in the alert head-free cat. Soc. Neurosci. Abstr. 12:458.

Munoz, D. P. and Guitton, D. (1989) Fixation and orientation control by the tecto-reticulo-spinal system in the cat whose head is unrestrained. Rev. Neurol. (Paris) 145:567–579.

Munoz, D. P. and Guitton, D. (1991) Control of orienting gaze shifts by the tectoreticulo-spinal system in the head-free cat. II. Sustained discharges during motor preparation and fixation. J. Neurophysiol. 66:1624–1641.

Munoz, D. P., Pelisson, D. and Guitton, D. (1991a) Movement of neural activity on the superior colliculus motor map during gaze shifts. Science 251:1358–1360.

Munoz, D. P., Guitton, D. and Pelisson, D. (1991b) Control of orienting gaze shifts by the tectoreticulospinal system in the head-free cat. III. Spatiotemporal characteristics of phasic motor discharges. J. Neurophysiol. 66:1642–1666.

Murata, K., Cramer, H. and Bach-y-Rita, P. (1965) Neuronal convergence of noxious, acoustic and visual stimuli in the visual cortex of the cat. J. Neurophysiol. 28:1123–1239.

Musil, S. Y. and Olson, C. R. (1988) Organization of cortical and subcortical projections to anterior cingulate cortex in the cat. J. Comp. Neurol. 272:203–218.

Nagata, T. and Kruger, L. (1979) Tactile neurons of the superior colliculus of the cat: Input and physiological properties. Brain Res. 174:19–37.

Naitoh, Y. and Eckert, R. (1969) Ciliary orientation: Controlled by cell membrane or by intracellular fibrils? Science 166:1633–1635.

Naitoh, Y. and Eckert, R. (1973) Sensory mechanisms in *Paramecium*. II. Ionic basis of the hyperpolarizing mechanoreceptor potential. J. Exp. Biol. 59:53–65.

Nashold, B. S., Jr., Wilson, W. P. and Slaughter, D. G. (1969) Sensations evoked by stimulation in the midbrain of man. J. Neurosurg. 30:14–24.

Natsoulas, T. and Dubanoski, R. (1964) Inferring the locus and orientation of the perceiver from responses to stimulation of the skin. Am. J. Psychol. 77:281–285.

Neafsey, E. J., Hurky-Gius, K. M. and Arvanitis, D. (1986) The topographical organization of neurons in the rat medial frontal, insular and olfactory cortex projecting to the solitary nucleus, olfactory bulb, periaqueductal gray and superior colliculus. Brain Res. 377: 261–270.

Necker, R. (1983) The problem of bimodal receptors: Responses to thermal stimuli. In *Multimodal Convergence in Sensory Systems*, E. Horn (ed.). New York: Fisher Verlag, pp. 1–16.

Nelson, J. S., Meredith, M. A. and Stein, B. E. (1989) Does an extraocular proprioceptive signal reach the superior colliculus? J. Neurophysiol. 62:1360–1374.

Newman, E. A. and Hartline, P. H. (1981) Integration of visual and infrared information in bimodal neurons of the rattlesnake optic tectum. Science 213:789–791.

Nickerson, R. S. (1973) Intersensory facilitation of reaction time: Energy summation or preparation enhancement? Psychol. Rev. 80:489–509.

Noda, H. (1981) Visual mossy fiber inputs to the flocculus of the monkey. Ann. N.Y. Acad. Sci. 374:465–475.

Norita, M. (1980) Neurons and synaptic patterns in the deep layers of the superior colliculus of the cat. A Golgi and electron microscopic study. J. Comp. Neurol. 190:29–48.

Northcutt, R. G. (1984) Evolution of the vertebrate central nervous system: Patterns and processes. Am. Zool. 24:701–716.

Northcutt, R. G. (1986) Evolution of the octavolateralis system: Evaluation and heuristic value of phylogenetic hypotheses. In *The Biology of Change in Otolaryngology*, R. Vanderwater and E. Rubel (eds.). New York: Excerpta Medica, pp 3–14.

Ogasawara, K., McHaffie, J. G. and Stein, B. E. (1984) Two visual systems in cat. J. Neurophysiol. 52:1226–1245.

Ogura, A. and Machemer, H. J. (1980) Distribution of mechanoreceptor channels in the *Paramecium* surface membrane. J. Comp. Physiol. [A] 135:233–242.

Olberg, R. M. and Willis, M. A. (1990) Pheromone-modulated optomotor response in male gypsy moths, *Lymantria dispar L.*: Direction selective visual interneurons in the ventral nerve cord. J. Comp. Physiol. 167:707–714.

Olivier, E., Chat, M. and Grantyn, A. (1991) Rostrocaudal and lateromedial density distributions of superior colliculus neurons projecting in the predorsal bundle and to the spinal cord—a retrograde HRP study in the cat. Exp. Brain Res. 87:268–282.

Olson, C. R. and Graybiel, A. M. (1987) Ectosylvian visual area of the cat: Location, retinotopic organization, and connections. J. Comp. Neurol. 261:277–294.

Palmer, A. R. and King, A. J. (1983) Monaural and binaural contributions to an auditory space map in the guinea-pig superior colliculus. In *Hearing: Physiological Bases and Psychophysics*, R. Klinhe and R. Hartmann (eds.). New York: Springer Verlag, pp. 230–236.

Palmer, A. R. and King, A. J. (1985) A monaural space map in the guinea-pig superior colliculus. Hearing Res. 17:267–280.

Passano, L. M. and McCullough, C. B. (1962). The light response and the rhythmic potentials of hydra. Proc. Natl. Acad. Sci. USA 48:1376–1382.

Pavlov, I. P. S. P. (1927) *Conditioned Reflexes*. Translated by G. V. Anrep. London: Oxford University Press.

Peck, C. K. (1987) Visual-auditory interactions in cat superior colliculus: Their role in control of gaze. Brain Res. 420:162–166.

Pelisson, D., Guitton, D. and Munoz, D. P. (1989) Compensatory eye and head movements generated by the cat following stimulation-induced perturbations in gaze position. Exp. Brain Res. 78:654–658.

Piaget, J. (1952) *The Origins of Intelligence in Children*, New York: International Universities Press.

Piaget, J. (1962) *Play, Dreams and Imitation in Childhood*, New York: W. W. Norton.

Pick, H. L., Jr. (1974) The visual coding on non-visual spatial information. In *Perception: Essays in Honor of James J. Gibson*, R. B. Macleod and H. L. Pick, Jr. (eds.). Ithaca: Cornell University Press.

Pick, H. L., Jr., Warren, D. H. and Hay, J. C. (1969) Sensory conflict in judgements of spatial direction. Percept. Psychophys. 6:203–205.

Poirier, L. J. and Bertrand, C. (1955) Experimental and anatomical investigation of the lateral spino-thalamic and spino-tectal tracts. J. Comp. Neurol. 102:745–758.

Poppell, E. Held, R. and Frost, D. (1973) Residual visual function after brain wounds involving the central visual pathways in man. Nature 243:295–296.

Posner, M. I., Nissen, M. J., and Klein, R. M. (1976) Visual dominance: An information-processing account of its origins and significance. Psychol. Rev. 83:157–171.

Precht, W. and Strata, P. (1980) On the pathway mediating optokinetic responses in vestibular neurons. Neuroscience 5:777–787.

Price, D. D. (1988) *Psychological and Neural Mechanisms of Pain*. New York: Raven.

Price, D. D., McHaffie, J. G. and Stein, B. E. (1992) The psychophysical attributes of heat-induced pain and their relationships to neural mechanisms. J. Cog. Neurosci. 4:1–14.

Rasmussen, K., Heym, J. and Jacobs, D. L. (1984) Activity of serotonin-containing neurons in nucleus centralis superior of freely moving cats. Exp. Neurol. 83:302–317.

Rauschecker, J. P. and Harris, L. R. (1989) Auditory and visual neurons in the cat's superior colliculus selective for the direction of apparent motion stimuli. Brain Res. 490:56–63.

Reale, R. A. and Imig, T. J. (1980) Tonotopic organization in auditory cortex of the cat. J. Comp. Neurol. 192:265–291.

Redgrave, P., Dean, P., Souki, W. and Lewis, G. (1981) Gnawing and changes in reactivity produced by microinjections of picrotoxin into the superior colliculus of rats. Psychopharmacology 75:198–203.

Redgrave, P., Odekunle, A. and Dean, P. (1986) Tectal cells of origin of predorsal bundle in rat: Location and segregation from ipsilateral descending pathway. Exp. Brain Res. 63:279–293.

Redgrave, P., Dean, P. and Westby, G. W. M. (1990) Organization of the crossed tecto-reticulo-spinal projection in rat. I. Anatomical evidence for separate output channels to the periabducens area and caudal medulla. Neuroscience 37:571–584.

Reyes, V., Henny, G. C., Baird, H., Wycis, H. T. and Spiegel, E. A. (1951) Localization of centripetal pathways of the human brain by recording evoked potentials. Trans. Am. Neurol. Assoc. 76:246–248.

Rhoades, R. W. (1980) The effects of neonatal enucleation upon the functional organization of the superior colliculus in the golden hamster. J. Physiol. 301:383–399.

Rhoades, R. W. and DellaCroce, D. R. (1980) Cells of origin of the tectospinal tract in the golden hamster: an anatomical and electrophysiological investigation. Exp. Neurol. 67:163–180.

Rhoades, R. W., DellaCroce, D. D. and Meadows, I. (1981) Reorganization of somatosensory input to superior colliculus in neonatally enucleated hamsters: Anatomical and electrophysiological experiments. J. Neurophysiol. 46:855–877.

Rhoades, R. W., Mooney, R. D. and Jacquin, M. R. (1983) Complex somatosensory receptive fields of neurons in the deep laminae of the hamster's superior colliculus. J. Neurosci. 3:1342–1354.

Rhoades, R. W., Mooney, R. D., Klein, B. G., Jacquin, M. F., Szczepanik, A. M. and Chiaia, N. L. (1987) The structural and functional characteristics of tectospinal neurons in the golden hamster. J. Comp. Neurol. 255:451–465.

Rhoades, R. W., Mooney, R. D., Rohrer, W. H., Nikoletseas, M. M. and Fish, S. E. (1989) Organization of the projection from the superficial to the deep layers of the hamster's superior colliculus as demonstrated by the anterograde transport of Phaseolus vulgaris leucoagglutinin. J. Comp. Neurol. 283:54–70.

Ritzmann, R. E., Pollack, A. J., Hudson, S. E. and Hyvonen, A. (1991) Convergence of multi-modal sensory signals at thoracic interneurons of the escape system of the cockroach, Periplaneta americana. Brain Res. 563:175–183.

Rizzolatti, G., Scandolara, C., Matelli, M. and Gentilucci, M. (1981a) Afferent properties of periarcuate neurons in macaque monkeys. I. Somatosensory responses. Behav. Brain Res. 2:125–146.

Rizzolatti, G., Scandolara, C., Matelli, M. and Gentilucci, M. (1981b) Afferent properties of periarcuate neurons in macaque monkeys. II. Visual responses. Behav. Brain Res. 2:147–163.

Robinson, D. A. (1972) Eye movements evoked by collicular stimulation in the alert monkey. Vision Res. 12:1796–1808.

Robinson, D. A. and Jarvis, C. D. (1974) Superior colliculus neurons studied during head and eye movements of the behaving monkey. J. Neurophysiol. 37:533–540.

Roe, A. W., Pallas, S. L., Hahm, J.-O. and Sur, M. (1990) A map of visual space induced in primary auditory cortex. Science 250:818–820.

Roll, R., Velay, J. L. and Roll, J. P. (1991) Eye and neck proprioceptive messages contribute to the spatial coding of retinal input in visually oriented activities. Exp. Brain Res. 85: 423–431.

Romer, A. S. (1970) The Vertebrate Body. Philadelphia: W. B. Saunders.

Room, P. and Groenewegen, H. J. (1986) Connections of the parahippocampal cortex. I. Cortical afferents. J. Comp. Neurol. 251:415–450.

Rose, S. A. (1990) Cross-modal transfer in human infants: What is being transferred? Ann. N.Y. Acad. Sci. 608:38–50.

Rosen, S. C., Weiss, K. R. and Kupfermann, I. (1982) Cross-modality sensory integration in the control of feeding in Aplysia. Behav. Neural Biol. 35:56–63.

Rosenquist, A. C. (1985) Connections of visual cortical areas in the cat. In Cerebral Cortex, Volume 3, A. Peter and E. G. Jones (eds.). New York: Plenum, pp. 81–118.

Roucoux, A. and Crommelinck, M. (1976) Eye movements evoked by superior colliculus stimulation in the alert cat. Brain Res. 106:349–363.

Rowell, C. H. R. and Reichert, H. (1986) Three descending interneurons reporting deviation from course in the locust. II. Physiology. J. Comp. Physiol. [A] 158:775–794.

Ryan, T. A. (1940) Interrelations of the sensory systems in perception. Psychol. Bull. 37:659–698.

Sahibzada, N., Dean, P. and Redgrave, P. (1986) Movements resembling orientation or avoidance elicited by electrical stimulation of the superior colliculus in rats. J. Neurosci. 6:723–733.

Sams, M., Aulanko, R., Hamalainen, M., Hari, R., Lounasmaa, O. V., Lu, S.-T. and Simola, J. (1991) Seeing speech: Visual information from lip movements modified activity in the human auditory cortex. Neurosci. Lett. 127:141–145.

Saraiva, P., Magalhaes-Castro, B., Magalhaes-Castro, H. and Torres, S. R. (1978) Electrophysiological aspects of the opossum superior colliculus. Corticotectal and tectotectal influences. In *Opossum Neurobiology*, C. E. Roche-Miranda and R. Lent (eds.). Rio de Janeiro: Academia Brasileiva de Ciencias, pp. 151–165.

Sato, T. (1989) Interactions of visual stimuli in the receptive fields of inferior temporal neurons in awake macaques. Exp. Brain Res. 77:23–30.

Satou, M., Matsushima, T., Takeuchi, H. and Ueda, K. (1985) Tongue-muscle-controlling motoneurons in the Japanese toad: Topography, morphology and neuronal pathways from the "snapping-evoking area" in the optic tectum. J. Comp. Physiol. [A] 157:717–737.

Schaefer, K. P. (1970) Unit analysis and electrical stimulation in the optic tectum of rabbits and cats. Brain Behav. Evol. 3:222–240.

Schiller, P. H. and Stryker, M. (1972) Single unit recording and stimulations in superior colliculus of the alert rhesus monkey. J. Neurophysiol. 35:915–924.

Schneider, G. E. (1967) Contrasting visuomotor function of tectum and cortex in the golden hamster. Psychol. Forsch. 31:52–62.

Schneider, G. E. (1969) Two visual systems: brain mechanisms for localization and discrimination are dissociated by tectal and cortical lesions. Science 163:895–902.

Schneider, J. S., Denaro, F. J. and Lidsky, T. I. (1982) Basal ganglia: Motor influences mediated by sensory interactions. Exp. Neurol. 77:534–543.

Segal, R. L. and Beckstead, R. M. (1984) The lateral suprasylvian corticotectal projection in cats. J. Comp. Neurol. 225:259–275.

Sesack, S. R., Deutch, A. Y., Roth, R. H. and Bunney, B. S. (1989) Topographical organization of the efferent projections of the medial prefrontal cortex in the rat: An anterograde tract-tracing study with *Phaeolus vulgaris* leucoagglutinin. J. Comp. Neurol. 290:213–242.

Shelton, B. R. and Searle, C. L. (1980) The influence of vision on the absolute identification of sound-source position. Percept. Psychophys. 28:589–596.

Sherman, S. M. (1974a) Visual fields of cats with cortical and tectal lesions. Science 185:355–357.

Sherman, S. M. (1974b) Permanence of visual perimetry deficits in monocularly and binocularly deprived cats. Brain Res. 73:491–501.

Sherrington, C. S. (1947) *The Integrative Action of the Nervous System* (2nd ed.). New Haven, Conn.: Yale University Press.

Shipley, T. (1980) *Sensory Integration in Children*. Springfield, Ill.: Charles C Thomas.

Siminoff, R., Schwassmann, O. and Kruger, L. (1966) An electrophysiological study of the visual projection to the superior colliculus of the rat. J. Comp. Neurol. 127:435–444.

Skinner, B. F. (1938) *The Behavior of Organisms: An Experimental Analysis.* New York: Appleton-Century-Crofts.

Solon, M. H. and Koopowitz, H. (1982) Multimodal interneurones in the polyclad flatworm, *Alloeplana californica.* J. Comp. Physiol. 147:171–178.

Sparks, D. L. (1975) Response properties of eye movement-related neurons in the monkey superior colliculus. Brain Res. 90:147–152.

Sparks, D. L. (1978) Functional properties of neurons in the monkey superior colliculus: Coupling of neuronal activity and saccadic onset. Brain Res. 156:1–16.

Sparks, D. L. (1989) The neural encoding of the location of targets for saccadic eye movements. J. Exp. Biol. 146:195–207.

Sparks, D. L. and Mays, L. E. (1983) Spatial localization of saccade targets. I. Compensation for stimulation-induced perturbations in eye position. J. Neurophysiol. 49:45–63.

Spelke, E. S. (1987) The development of intermodal perception. In *Handbook of Infant Perception, Vol. 2,* P. Salapatek and L. Cohen (eds.). New York: Academic, pp. 233–273.

Spiegel, E. A., Kletzkin, M. S. and Szekely, E. G. (1954) Pain reactions upon stimulation of the tectum mesencephali. J. Neuropathol. Exp. Neurol. 13:212–220.

Spinelli, D. N., Starr, A. and Barrett, T. W. (1968) Auditory specificity in unit recordings from cat's visual cortex. Exp. Neurol. 22:75–84.

Sprague, J. M. (1963) Corticofugal projections to the superior colliculus in the cat. Anat. Rec. 145:288.

Sprague, J. M. (1966a) Interaction of cortex and the superior colliculus in mediation of visually guided behavior in the cat. Science 153:1544–1546.

Sprague, J. M. (1966b) Visual, acoustic, and somesthetic deficits in the cat after cortical and midbrain lesions. In *The Thalamus,* D. D. Purpura and M. Yahr (eds.). New York: Columbia University Press, pp. 391–417.

Sprague, J. M. and Meikle, T. H. Jr. (1965) The role of the superior colliculus in visually guided behavior. Exp. Neurol. 11:115–146.

Springer, A. D., Easter, S. S., Jr. and Agranoff, B. W. (1977) The role of the optic tectum in various visually mediated behaviors of goldfish. Brain Res. 128:393–404.

Stein, B. E. (1978) Nonequivalent visual, auditory and somatic corticotectal influences in cat. J. Neurophysiol. 41:55–64.

Stein, B. E. (1981) Organization of the rodent superior colliculus: Some comparisons with other mammals. Behav. Brain Res. 3:175–188.

Stein, B. E. (1984a) Multimodal representation in the superior colliculus and optic tectum. In *Comparative Neurology of the Optic Tectum,* H. Vanegas (ed.). New York: Plenum, pp. 819–841.

Stein, B. E. (1984b) Development of the superior colliculus. Annu. Rev. Neurosci. 7:95–125.

Stein, B. E. (1988a) Superior colliculus-mediated visual behaviors in cat and the concept of two corticotectal systems. In *Progress in Brain Research, Vol. 75,* T. P. Hicks and G. Benedek (eds.). New York: Elsevier, pp. 37–53.

Stein, B. E. (1988b) Concepts of brain evolution. Behav. Brain Sci. 11:100–101.

Stein, B. E. and Arigbede, M. O. (1972) Unimodal and multimodal response properties of neurons in the cat's superior colliculus. Exp. Neurol. 36:179–196.

Stein, B. E. and Clamann, H. P. (1981) Control of pinna movements and sensorimotor register in cat superior colliculus. Brain Behav. Evol. 19:180–192.

Stein, B. E. and Dixon, J. P. (1978) Superior colliculus neurons respond to noxious stimuli. Brain Res. 158:65–73.

Stein, B. E. and Dixon, J. P. (1979) Properties of superior colliculus neurons in the golden hamster. J. Comp. Neurol. 183:269–284.

Stein, B. E. and Gaither, N. (1981) Sensory representation in reptilian optic tectum: Some comparisons with mammals. J. Comp. Neurol. 202:69–87.

Stein, B. E. and Gaither, N. (1983) Receptive field properties in reptilian optic tectum: Some comparisons with mammals. J. Neurophysiol. 50:102–124.

Stein, B. E. and Gallagher, H. (1981) Maturation of cortical control over superior colliculus cells in cat. Brain Res. 223:429–435.

Stein, B. E. and Meredith, M. A. (1990) Multisensory integration: Neural and behavioral solutions for dealing with stimuli from different sensory modalities. Ann. N.Y. Acad. Sci. 608:51–70.

Stein, B. E. and Meredith, M. A. (1991) Functional organization of the superior colliculus. In *The Neural Bases of Visual Function*, A. G. Leventhal (ed.). Hampshire, U.K.: Macmillan, pp. 85–110.

Stein, B. E., Labos, E. and Kruger, L. (1973) Sequence of changes in properties of neurons of superior colliculus of the kitten during maturation. J. Neurophysiol. 36:667–679.

Stein, B. E., Goldberg, S. J. and Clamann, H. P. (1976a) The control of eye movements by the superior colliculus in the alert cat. Brain Res. 118:469–474.

Stein, B. E., Magalhaes-Castro, B. and Kruger, L. (1976b) Relationship between visual and tactile representation in cat superior colliculus. J. Neurophysiol. 39:401–419.

Stein, B. E., Clamann, H. P. and Goldberg, S. J. (1980) Superior colliculus: Control of eye movements in neonatal kittens. Science 210:78–80.

Stein, B. E., Spencer, R. F. and Edwards, S. B. (1982) Efferent projections of the neonatal superior colliculus: Extraoculomotor-related brain stem structures. Brain Res. 239:17–28.

Stein, B. E., Spencer, R. F. and Edwards, S. B. (1983) Corticotectal and corticothalamic efferent projections of SIV somatosensory cortex in cat. J. Neurophysiol. 50:896–909.

Stein, B. E., Huneycutt, W. S. and Meredith, M. A. (1988) Neurons and behavior: The same rules of multisensory integration apply. Brain Res. 448:355–358.

Stein, B. E., Meredith, M. A., Huneycutt, W. S. and McDade, L. (1989a) Behavioral indices of multisensory integration: Orientation to visual cues is affected by auditory stimuli. J. Cog. Neurosci. 1:12–24.

Stein, B. E., Price, D. D. and Gazzaniga, M. S. (1989b) Pain perception in a man with total corpus callosum transection. Pain 38:51–56.

Stein, B. E., Meredith, M. A. and Wallace, M. T. (1993) Nonvisual responses of visually-responsive neurons. In *Progress in Brain Research: The Visually Responsive Neuron: From Basic Neurophysiology to Behavior*, T. P. Hicks, S. Molotchnikoff and T. Ono (eds.). Amsterdam: Elsevier, in press.

Stevens, S. S. (1975) *Psychophysics: Introduction to Its Perceptual, Neural and Social Prospects*. New York: Wiley.

Straschill, M. and Hoffmann, K.-P. (1970) Activity of movement sensitive neurons of the cat's tectum opticum during spontaneous eye movements. Exp. Brain Res. 11:318–326.

Straschill, M. and Schick, F. (1977) Discharges of superior colliculus neurons during head and eye movements of the alert cat. Exp. Brain Res. 27:131–141.

Strausfeld, N. J. and Bassemir, U. K. (1985) Lobula plate and ocellar interneurons converge on a cluster of descending neurons leading to neck and leg motor neuropil in *Calliphora erythrocephala.* Cell Tissue Res. 240:617–640.

Strausfeld, N. J., Bassemir, U., Singh, R. N. and Bacon, J. P. (1984) Organizational principles of outputs from dipteran brains. J. Insect Physiol. 30:73–93.

Strecker, R. E., Steinfels, G. F., Abercrombie, E. D. and Jacobs, B. L. (1985) Caudate unit activity in freely moving cats: Effects of phasic auditory and visual stimuli. Brain Res. 329:350–353.

Sumby, W. H. and Pollack, I. (1954) Visual contribution to speech intelligibility in noise. J. Acoust. Soc. Am. 26:212–215.

Syka, S. and Radil-Weiss, T. (1971) Electrical stimulation of the tectum in freely moving cats. Brain Res. 28:567–572.

Tautz, J. (1987) Interneurons in the tritocerebrum of the crayfish. Brain Res. 407:230–239.

Tautz, J. and Sandeman, D. C. (1980) the detection of waterborne vibration by sensory hairs on the chelae of the crayfish. J. Exp. Biol. 88:351–356.

Tawil, R. N., Saade, N., Bitar, M. and Jabbur, S. J. (1983) Polysensory interactions on single neurons of cat inferior colliculus. Brain Res. 269:149–152.

Terashima, S.-I. and Goris, R. C. (1975) Tectal organization of pit viper infrared reception. Brain Res. 83:490–494.

Thompson, G. C. and Masterton, R. B. (1978) Brain stem auditory pathways involved in reflexive head orientation to sound. J. Neurophysiol. 41:1183–1202.

Thurlow, W. R. and Rosenthal, T. M. (1976) Further study of existence regions for the "ventriloquism effect." J. Am. Audiol. Soc. 1:280–286.

Tiao, Y.-C. and Blakemore, C. (1976) Functional organization in the superior colliculus of the golden hamster. J. Comp. Neurol. 168:483–506.

Tokunaga, A., Sugitz, S. and Otani, K. (1984) Auditory and non-auditory subcortical afferents to the inferior colliculus in the rat. J. Hirnforsch. 35:461–472.

Toldi, J., Feher, O., and Feuer, L. (1984) Dynamic interactions of evoked potentials in a polysensory cortex of the cat. Neuroscience 13:945–952.

Tortelly, A., Reinoso-Suarez, F. and Llamas, A. (1980) Projections from non-visual cortical areas to the superior colliculus demonstrated by retrograde transport of HRP in the cat. Brain Res. 188:543–549.

Traub, B. and Elepfandt, A. (1990) Sensory neglect in a frog: Evidence for early evolution of attentional processes in vertebrates. Brain Res. 530:105–107.

Tricas, T. C. and Highstein, S. M. (1990) Visually mediated inhibition of lateral line primary afferent activity by the octavolateralis efferent system during predation in the free-swimming toadfish, *Opsanus tau.* Exp. Brain Res. 83:233–236.

Turkewitz, G. and Mellon, R. C. (1989) Dynamic organization of intersensory function. Can. J. Psychol. 43:286–307.

Vaadia, E., Benson, D. A., Heinz, R. D. and Goldstein, M. H. (1986) Unit study of monkey frontal cortex: Active localization of auditory and of visual stimuli. J. Neurophysiol. 56:934–952.

Vanegas, H., Ebbesson, S. O. E. and Laufer, M. (1984) Morphological aspects of the teleostean optic tectum. In *Comparative Neurology of the Optic Tectum*, H. Vanegas (ed.). New York: Plenum, pp. 93–120.

Van Gisbergen, J. A. M., Van Opstal, A. J. and Tax, A. A. M. (1987) Collicular ensemble coding of saccades based on vector summation. Neuroscience 21:541–555.

Van Hoesen, G. W. (1982) The parahippocampal gyrus. New observations regarding its cortical connections in the monkey. Trends Neurosci. 5:345–350.

Van Houten, J. and Preston, R. R. (1988) Chemokinesis. In *Paramecium*, H.-D. Gortz (ed.). Berlin: Springer-Verlag, pp. 282–300.

Vidal, P.-P., May, P. J. and Baker, R. (1988) Synaptic organization of the tectal-facial pathways in the cat. I. Synaptic potentials following collicular stimulation. J. Neurophysiol. 60:769–797.

Vincent, S. B. (1912) The function of the vibrissae in the behavior of the white rat. Behav. Monogr. 1:1–81.

Volchan, E., Rocha-Miranda, C. E., Lent, R. and Gawryszewski, L. G. (1978) The retinotopic organization of the superior colliculus in the opossum (Didelphis Marsupialis Aurita). In *Opossum Neurobiology*. Academia Brasileira de Ciencias, Rio de Janeiro.

von Hornbostel, E. M. (1938) The unity of the senses. In *A Sourcebook of Gestalt Psychology*, W. D. Ellis (ed.). New York: Harcourt Brace, pp. 211–216.

Wade, N. J. and Day, R. H. (1968) Apparent head position as a basis for a visual aftereffect of prolonged head tilt. Percep. Psychophys. 3:324–326.

Waespe, W. and Henn, V. (1979) Motion information in the vestibular nuclei of alert monkeys: visual and vestibular inputs vs. optomotor output. Prog. Brain Res. 50:683–693.

Waespe, W. and Henn, V. (1981) Visual-vestibular interaction in the flocculus of the alert monkey. II. Purkinje cell activity. Exp. Brain Res. 43:349–360.

Waespe, W., Buttner, U. and Henn, V. (1981) Input-output activity of the primate flocculus during visual-vestibular interaction. Ann. N.Y. Acad. Sci. 374:491–503.

Walker, A. E. (1942) The relief of pain by mesencephalic tractotomy. Arch. Neurol. Psychiatry 48:865–883.

Walker, A. E. (1943) Central representation of pain. Res. Publ. Assoc. Res. Nerv. Ment. Dis. 23:63–85.

Wallace, M. T., Meredith, M. A. and Stein, B. E. (1991) Cortical convergence on multisensory output neurons of cat superior colliculus. Soc. Neurosci. Abstr. 17:1379.

Wallace, M. T., Meredith, M. A. and Stein, B. E. (1992) The integration of multiple sensory inputs in cat cortex. Exp. Brain Res., in press.

Wallace, S. F., Rosenquist, A. C. and Sprague, J. M. (1989) Recovery from cortical blindness mediated by destruction of nontectotectal fibers in the commissure of the superior colliculus in the cat. J. Comp. Neurol. 284:429–450.

Wallace, S. F., Rosenquist, A. C. and Sprague, J. M. (1990) Ibotenic acid lesions of the lateral substantia nigra restore visual orientation in the hemianopic cat. J. Comp. Neurol. 296:222–252.

Wallach, H. and Averback, E. (1955) On memory modalities. Am. J. Psychol. 58:249–257.

Walter, G. W. (1964) The convergence and interaction of visual, auditory and tactile responses in human non-specific cortex. Ann. N.Y. Acad. Sci. 122:320–361.

Warren, D. H., Welch, R. B. and McCarthy, T. J. (1981) The role of visual-auditory "compellingness" in the ventriloquism effect: Implications for transitivity among the spatial senses. Percept. Psychophys. 30:557–564.

Watanabe, J. and Iwai, E. (1991) Neuronal activity in visual, auditory and polysensory areas of the monkey temporal cortex during visual fixation task. Brain Res. Bull. 26: 583–592.

Weber, J. T., Martin, G. G., Behan, M., Huerta, M. F. and Harting, J. K. (1979) The precise origin of the tectospinal pathway in three common laboratory animals: A study using the horseradish peroxidase method. Neurosci. Lett. 11:121–127.

Webster, K. E. (1974) Changing concepts of the organization of the central visual pathways in birds. In *Essays on the Nervous System*, R. Bellairs and E. G. Gray (eds.). Oxford: Clarendon Press, pp. 258–298.

Weiskrantz, L. (1961) Encephalisation and the scotoma. In *Current Problems in Animal Behavior*, W. H. Thorpe and O. L. Zangwill (eds.), Cambridge: Cambridge University Press, pp. 30–58.

Weiskrantz, L., Warrington, E. K., Sanders, M. D. and Marshall, J. (1974) Visual capacity in the hemianopic field following a restricted occipital ablation. Brain 97:709–728.

Welch, R. B. and Warren, D. H. (1980) Immediate perceptual response to intersensory discrepancy. Psychol. Bull. 88:638–667.

Welch, R. B. and Warren, D. H. (1986) Intersensory interactions. In *Handbook of Perception and Human Performance, Volume I: Sensory Processes and Perception*, K. R. Boff, L. Kaufman and J. P. Thomas (eds.). New York: Wiley, pp. 25-1–25-36.

Weldon, D. A. and Best, P. J. (1992) Changes in sensory responsivity in deep layer neurons of the superior colliculus of behaving rats. Behav. Brain Res. 47:97–101.

Werner, C. and Himstedt, W. (1985) Mechanism of head orientation during prey capture in salamander (*Salamandra salamandra L.*). Zool. J. Physiol. 89:359–368.

Wespic, J. G. (1966) Multimodal sensory activation of cells in the magnocellular medial geniculate nucleus. Exp. Neurol. 15:299–318.

West, C. K. and Michael, R. P. (1990) Responses of units in the mesolimbic system to olfactory and somatosensory stimuli: Modulation of sensory input by ventral tegmental stimulation. Brain Res. 532:307–316.

Westby, G. W. M., Keay, K. A., Redgrave, P., Dean, P. and Bannister, M. (1990) Output pathways from the rat superior colliculus mediating approach and avoidance have different sensory properties. Exp. Brain Res. 81:626–638.

Wickelgren, B. G. (1971) Superior colliculus: Some receptive field properties of bimodally responsive cells. Science 173:69–71.

Wickelgren, B. G. and Sterling, P. (1969) Influence of visual cortex on receptive fields in the superior colliculus of the cat. J. Neurophysiol. 32:16–23.

Wiersma, C. A. G. (1947) Giant nerve fiber system of the crayfish. A contribution of comparative physiology of synapse. J. Neurophysiol. 10:23–38.

Wiersma, C. A. G. and Mill, P. J. (1965) "Descending" neuronal units in the commissure of the crayfish central nervous system and their integration of visual, tactile and proprioceptive stimuli. J. Comp. Neurol. 125:67–94.

Willis, M. A. and Carde, R. T. (1990) Pheromone-modulated optomotor response in male gypsy moths, *Lymantria dispar L.*: Upwind flight in a pheromone plume in different wind velocities. J. Comp. Physiol. [A] 167:699–706.

Wilson, J. S., Hull, C. D. and Buchwald, N. A. (1983) Intracellular studies of the convergence of sensory input on caudate neurons of cat. Brain Res. 270:197–208.

Wine, J. J. and Krasne, F. B. (1972) The organization of escape behaviour in the crayfish. J. Exp. Biol. 56:1–18.

Wise, L. Z. and Irvine, D. R. F. (1983) Auditory response properties of neurons in deep layers of cat superior colliculus. J. Neurophysiol. 49:674–685.

Wise, L. Z. and Irvine, D. R. F. (1985) Topographic organization of interaural intensity difference sensitivity in deep layers of cat superior colliculus: Implications for auditory spatial representation. J. Neurophysiol. 54:185–211.

Withington-Wray, D. J., Dhanjal, S. S., Binns, K. E. and Keating, M. J. (1989) The development of a map of auditory space in the superior colliculus—prevention by rearing in an environment of continuous omnidirectional auditory stimulation. Neurosci. Lett. Suppl. 36:S6.

Withington-Wray, D. J., Binns, K. E. and Keating, M. J. (1990a) The maturation of the superior collicular map of auditory space in the guinea pig is disrupted by developmental visual deprivation. Eur. J. Neurosci. 2:682–692.

Withington-Wray, D. J., Binns, K. E., Dhanjal, S. S., Brickley, S. G. and Keating, M. J. (1990b) The maturation of the collicular map of auditory space in the guinea pig is disrupted by developmental auditory deprivation. Eur. J. Neurosci. 2:693–703.

Wood, D. (1970) Electrophysiological studies of the protozoan *Stentor coeruleus*. J. Neurobiol. 1:363–377.

Woolsey, C. N. (1981) *Cortical Sensory Organization, Vol. 2: Multiple Visual Areas*. Clifton, N.J.: Humana Press.

Wurtz, R. H. and Goldberg, M. E. (1971) Superior colliculus cell responses related to eye movements in awake monkeys. Science 171:82–84.

Yen, C. T. and Blum, P. S. (1984) Response properties and functional organization of neurons in midline region of medullary reticular formation of cats. J. Neurophysiol. 52:951–979.

Zarzeki, P., Blum, P. S., Bakker, D. A. and Herman, D. (1983) Convergence of sensory inputs on projection neurons of somatosensory cortex: vestibular, neck, head and forelimb inputs. Exp. Brain Res. 50:408–414.

Zihl, J. (1980) "Blindsight": Improvement of visually guided eye movements by systematic practice in patients with cerebral blindness. Neuropsychologia 18:71–77.

Zimmermann, M. (1976) Neurophysiology of nociception. In *International Review of Physiology, Neurophysiology II, Volume 10*, R. Porter (ed.). Baltimore: University Park Press, pp. 179–221.

Author Index

Subject Index

Note: Italic *f* after a page number indicates a figure, *t* indicates a table.

premotor (presaccadic) burst, 53, 57, 57f
  and saccadic amplitude, 53, 147
  and saccadic latency, 53, 56
  and saccadic velocity, 53, 147
Movement field, 53, 54f
Multisensory convergence
  in advanced invertebrates, 27–29
  in anterior ectosylvian cortex, 170–171, 171f
  in auditory system, 7
  frequency, in superior colliculus, 117–118, 118f
  general, 2, 14–15, 107–108, 108f, 117–118 (*see also* Synesthesia)
  in insects, 29–32
  in integrated maps, 112–115
  in intraparietal cortex, 36, 170
  in optic tectum, 118
  in primary visual cortex, 169
  in primitive invertebrates, 25–27
  in somatosensory system, 6
  in superior colliculus, 117–122, 118f, 120–121f
  in temporal cortex, 36, 170
  in unicellular organisms, 22–25
  in unimodal maps, 108, 114
  in vertebrates, 33–37
  in vestibular system, 6–7
  in visual system, 6–7
Multisensory integration
  comparison with unimodal integration, 142–143, 144f
  in crustaceans, 27–29
  depression (*see* response depression)
  effect of experience on, 123
  effects on orientation behaviors, 148–156, 148–150f, 152–154f, 156f
    and stimulus spatial coincidence, 149, 149f, 153f
    and stimulus spatial disparity, 151–153, 152–153f
    and stimulus spatial resolution, 153–154, 154f
  effects on premotor discharges, 147–148
  effects on stimulus salience, 147
  enhancement (*see* response enhancement)
  formula for calculating magnitude, 125
  in *Hermissenda crassicornis*, 32–33
  inhibition, 137–140
  in insects, 29–32
  and inverse effectiveness, 143–146, 145f
  NMDA involvement, 144

and oculographic perceptual effects, 6
physiological-behavioral correlates, 153, 155–156, 156f
in Platyhelminthes (flatworms), 26–27
response depression, 123, 128–134, 128f, 172, 172f
response enhancement, 123–129, 124f, 126f, 127f, 143, 171–172, 172f
rules, 116
  inverse of unimodal effectiveness, 143–146, 145f, 171
  multiplicative effects, 142–143, 144f
  receptive field properties, preservation of, 140–142, 142f
  spatial, 129–134, 131–133f, 160, 171, 171f
  temporal, 134–140, 134–141f, 171
survival value of, 146, 148f
in unicellular organisms, 24–25
and vestibulo-auditory perceptual effects, 5
and vestibulo-oculomotor perceptual effects, 6
and vestibulo-visual perceptual effects, 4–7, 10–11, 31–32
and visual-auditory perceptual effects, 6, 8
and visual-proprioceptive perceptual effects, 6, 11, 12
and visual-somatosensory perceptual effects, 16, 18
Multisensory map, 114–115, 112f
Multisensory-multimotor map, 115–116
Multisensory receptive fields. *See also* Multisensory convergence; Multisensory integration; Sensory maps alignment
  development of, 123–124, 164–167, 165f, 173
  disruption of, 134, 135f, 157–166, 159f, 162f, 163f
  general, 112, 131f, 156, 169–173
  maintenance of, 157–164, 159–163f
cortical neurons, 169–172, 171f, 172f
examples of, 114f, 131–135f, 140f, 156f, 165f, 171–172f
mapping convention, 113f
properties of, 118–119, 129–130, 140–142, 142f
size, 111, 118
Nociception, 77–82, 95. *See also* Sensory maps
Nociceptive-specific. *See* Nociception
Nucleus sagulum, 46

Occlusion, 143, 144

Oculogravic illusion, 6. *See also* Vestibular system, effects on vision

Optic tectum, 41, 59–61, 96–98. *See also* Superior colliculus; Tectum

Orienting behavior, 39, 40*f*, 49, 51, 62–63, 62*f*, 99–100, 149–149, 148*f*, 149*f*, 155, 156*f*

Owl. *See* Birds

Pain. *See* Nociception

Paramecium. *See* Unicellular organisms

Pavlovian conditioning, 33

Perihypoglossal nucleus, 47

Perimetry, 66, 68

Periolivary nucleus, 46

Platyhelminthes, 26–27

Point image, 89, 91

Posterior commissure, nucleus, 46

Postexcitatory inhibition, 137

Premotor, 53, 56–58, 115–116. *See also* Multisensory integration, effect on premotor discharges; Superior colliculus

Preparation enhancement, 7–8

Presaccadic. *See* Gaze; Premotor; Saccades; Superior colliculus, visuomotor involvement

Primary orbital position, 161

Primates, 82, 87–88, 93, 161–163, 162–163*f*, 170

Primitive unity hypothesis, 11–12, 21, 24

Primordial organism, 21, 24, 36

Proprioception, 5, 6. *See also* Somatosensory system; Vestibular system

Protist. *See* Unicellular organisms

Rabbit, 93, 102

Rattlesnake, 94, 97

Rays, 103

Reaction time, 7, 8

Receptive field properties. *See also* Multisensory receptive fields
  auditory, 71–73, 73*f*
    best areas, 72–73, 73*f*, 92, 162–164
    binaural properties, 72–73
    and ear movement, 163–164
    latency, 135
  nociceptive, 78–80, 79*f*, 95
  somatosensory, 74–76, 75*f*, 162
    latency, 135
  visual, 64–66, 65–66*f*, 141–142, 141*f*
    latency, 135

Reptiles, 96–97, 103–104

Reticular activating system, 35

Retina, 44, 46

Rodents, 62–63, 76, 80, 88, 93, 94, 102, 166–167

Saccades, 52, 56. *See also* Eye movements

Salamander, 166

Sensory maps, 53, 83–84. *See also* Multisensory receptive fields; Superior colliculus
  alignment, with motor maps, 100–102, 101*f*
  auditory, 83, 92–93, 93*f*,112*f*, 161, 164–167
    effects of altered development 164–166, 165*f*
    effects of dark rearing, 166
    effects of ear movements, 163, 163*f*
    effects of eye movements (*see* Compensation; Multisensory receptive fields, alignment)
    tonotopic, 72, 92
  multisensory, 111–115, 112–113*f*
    active misalignments, 111, 157–163
    alignment, 90–91, 97–98, 111–112
    developmental misalignments, 164–167
  in nonmammals, 96–98
  somatosensory, 90–92, 91*f*, 95, 96, 112*f*
    effects of altered development, 166–167
    nociceptive, 95, 95*f*
    vibrissae (whiskers), 94–95, 94*f*
  visual
    deep layer, 88–92, 89*f*, 112*f*
    effects of eye movements, 158–159, 159*f*
    superficial layer, 87–88, 88*f*, 164–166

Sensory neglect, 62

Sensory properties. *See* Receptive field properties

Somatosensory system
  afferents to superior colliculus, 43*t*, 45–46
  cortex, 35, 43*f*, 45–46, 76, 120, 121*f*, 170
  corticotectal projection, 43*f*, 45–46, 76, 120, 121*f*, 170
  and cross-modal transfer, 15, 16*f*
  dorsal column nuclei, 46
  effects on vision, 31
  lateral cervical nucleus, 46
  map in superior colliculus, 90–92, 91*f*, 94–95, 94–95*f*, 96, 97*f*, 112*f*
  multisensory convergence in, 6, 34
  nociception, 77
  properties (*see* Receptive field properties)
  receptor categories, 74–75
  spinal cord dorsal horn, 46

trigeminal complex, 46
ventrobasal complex, 35
Somatosensory properties. *See* Receptive
field properties
Somatotopic map, 90, 96. *See also* Sensory
maps, somatosensory
Sound
latency for superior colliculus response,
135
velocity (in air), 135
Spinal cord dorsal horn, 46
Spinothalamic pathway, 77
Sprague effect, 66–69, 67*f*
State-dependent effects, 18, 44
Summation, 145
Superior colliculus
afferents
motor, 46–47, 43*f,t*
sensory, 43–46, 43*f,t*
anatomy, 41, 47, 42*f*
efferents, 47–49, 48*f*, 57, 59, 121–122, 121*f*
ascending projection, 47
contralateral descending (crossed
descending, tecto-reticulospinal tract,
or predorsal bundle), 47, 48, 121*f*, 122
intercollicular commissure, 47, 48, 67
ipsilateral descending, 47, 82
function, 39–40, 40*f*, 44, 62, 64–69, 66*f*,
68*f*, 74–75, 80–82, 81*f*, 85, 102 (*see also*
Two visual systems)
orienting behavior, 39, 40*f*, 49, 51, 62–
63, 62*f*, 99–100, 148*f*, 149, 149*f*, 155,
156*f*
withdrawal/avoidance behavior, 80–83,
81*f*, 102–104
intercollicular commissure, 47, 48, 67
interneurons, 47
laminar pattern, 41–42, 42*f*
superficial-deep dichotomy, 42, 44–45,
63
lesions of, 62–63, 66, 68, 74, 76–77,
neuronal morphology, 47
sensorimotor transformation, 56–59, 85,
116, 148
sensory properties (*see* Receptive field
properties)
tecto-reticulospinal neurons, 48, 49
visuomotor involvement, 51–59, 147
visual grasp reflex, 52
Synesthesia, 9–10

Tectum(al), 41, 65. *See also* Optic tectum;
Superior colliculus
Tectospinal, 41, 49

Thalamic reticular nucleus, 46
Thalamus, 35, 58, 79
Tonotopic. *See* Sensory maps
Trapezoid body, 46
Trigeminal nucleus, 46
Two visual systems, 61–63

Unicellular organisms, 22–25, 37
Unimodal integration, compared with
multisensory integration, 142–143, 144*f*
Unity of the senses. *See* Primitive unity
hypothesis

Ventriloquism effect, 3. *See also* Intersensory bias
Ventrobasal complex, 35
Vestibular system, 4, 5
effects on audition, 5
effects on gaze, 6
effects on vision, 4–7, 10–11, 31–32
gravity, 5, 6
in primitive animals, 27
Vibrissae. *See* Whiskers
Vision/visual system
afferents to superior colliculus, 43–45, 43*t*
alterations in perception, 5, 10
cortex, 18, 63, 66, 66*f*, 68, 69
corticotectal, 41, 44, 65–69
effects on auditory perception, 6, 8
effects on somatosensory perception, 16,
18
evolutionary trends, 59–61
gaze, 6, 7
lateral geniculate nucleus, 35
lesion and deficits, 60, 62–63, 66–69
map in superior colliculus, 52
deep layer, 88–92, 89*f*, 112*f*
superficial layer, 87–88, 88*f*
multisensory convergence in, 6–7, 34, 35,
and proprioception, 6, 11, 12
response properties (*see* Receptive field
properties)
Visual-analogue scale, 17
Visual grasp reflex, 52
Visual neglect, 62, 62*f*, 66, 67*f*, 68, 68*f*
Visual properties. *See* Receptive field properties
Visuotopic, 87, 96. *See also* Sensory maps,
visual

Whiskers (vibrissae), 76, 94–95, 94*f*, 102
Wide dynamic range. *See* Nociception

Zona incerta, 46

Printed in the United States
by Baker & Taylor Publisher Services